Manual of Emergency
Airway Management

Manual of Emergency Airway Management

Editor-in-Chief

Ron M. Walls, M.D., F.R.C.P.C., F.A.C.E.P.
Chairman, Department of Emergency Medicine
Brigham and Women's Hospital
Associate Professor of Medicine
Division of Emergency Medicine
Harvard Medical School
Boston, Massachusetts

Contributing Editors

Robert C. Luten, M.D.
Professor of Emergency Medicine and Pediatrics
University of Florida
Jacksonville, Florida

Michael F. Murphy, M.D., F.R.C.P.
Departments of Emergency Medicine and Anaesthesiology
Queen Elizabeth II Health Sciences Centre
Dalhousie University
Halifax, Nova Scotia

Robert E. Schneider, M.D.
Department of Emergency Medicine
Carolinas Medical Center
Charlotte, North Carolina

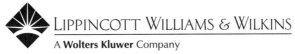

LIPPINCOTT WILLIAMS & WILKINS
A **Wolters Kluwer** Company
Philadelphia · Baltimore · New York · London
Buenos Aires · Hong Kong · Sydney · Tokyo

Acquisitions Editor: Elizabeth Greenspan
Developmental Editor: Sonya L. Seigafuse
Production Editor: Jeff Somers
Manufacturing Manager: Kevin Watt
Cover Design: Mark Lerner
Compositor: Circle Graphics
Printer: Maple Press

© 2000 by Ron M. Walls, M. D.
Published by Lippincott Williams & Wilkins
530 Walnut Street
Philadelphia, PA 19106 USA
LWW.com

Library of Congress Cataloging-in-Publication Data

Manual of emergency airway management / editor-in chief, Ron M. Walls ;
contributing editors, Robert C. Luten, Michael F. Murphy, Robert E. Schneider.
    p. ; cm.
  Includes bibliographical references and index.
  ISBN 0-7817-2616-6 (alk. paper)
  1. Respiratory emergencies—Handbooks, manuals, etc. 2. Respiratory intensive
care—Handbooks, manuals, etc. 3. Airway (Medicine)—Handbooks, manuals, etc. I.
Walls, Ron M.
  [DNLM: 1. Airway Obstruction—therapy—Handbooks. 2. Emergency
Treatment—Handbooks. 3. Intubation, Intratracheal—Handbooks. WF 39 H236 2000]
RC735.R48 H36 2000
616.2′00425—dc21

00-022742

10 9 8 7 6 5 4 3 2 1

Contents

Appendix

Contributing Authors

Diane M. Birnbaumer, M.D.   *Associate Professor of Medicine, UCLA School of Medicine, Los Angeles, California 90509; Associate Residency Director, Department of Emergency Medicine, Harbor UCLA Medical Center, 1000 West Carson Street, Box 21, Torrance, California 90509*

Michael A. Gibbs, M.D., F.A.C.E.P.   *Residency Program Director, Medical Director of Air-Medical Services, Department of Emergency Medicine, Carolinas Medical Center, 1000 Blythe Boulevard, Charlotte, North Carolina 28203*

Robert C. Luten, M.D.   *Professor of Emergency Medicine and Pediatrics, University of Florida, 655 West 8th Street, Jacksonville, Florida 32209*

Gregory W. Murphy, B.Sc., R.R.T.   *Hospital Clinical Consultant, Respiratory Group, Mallinckrodt Incorporated, 675 McDonnell Boulevard, St. Louis, Missouri 63134*

Michael F. Murphy, M.D., F.R.C.P.C.   *Associate Professor, Departments of Emergency Medicine and Anaesthesiology, Queen Elizabeth II Health Sciences Centre, Dalhousie University, Halifax, Nova Scotia*

Charles V. Pollack, Jr., M.A., M.D., F.A.C.E.P.   *Associate Clinical Professor of Surgery, Department of Emergency Medicine, University of Arizona College of Medicine, Tucson, Arizona; Department of Emergency Medicine, Maricopa Medical Center and Arizona Heart Hospital, Phoenix, Arizona 85008*

John C. Sakles, M.D.   *Assistant Professor, Department of Emergency Medicine, University of Cincinnati College of Medicine, 231 Bethesda Avenue, Cincinnati, Ohio 45140-0769; Attending Physician, Department of Emergency Medicine, University of Cincinnati Medical Center, 234 Goodman Street, Cincinnati, Ohio 45267-1000*

Robert E. Schneider, M.D.   *Academic Faculty, Department of Emergency Medicine, Carolinas Medical Center, 1000 Blythe Boulevard, P.O. Box 32861, Charlotte, North Carolina 28232*

Robert J. Vissers, M.D., F.A.C.E.P., F.R.C.P.C.   *Assistant Professor, Department of Emergency Medicine, University of North Carolina School of Medicine, 101 Manning Drive, CB # 7594, Chapel Hill, North Carolina 27599-7594*

Ron M. Walls, M.D., F.R.C.P.C., F.A.C.E.P.   *Chairman, Department of Emergency Medicine, Brigham and Women's Hospital; Associate Professor of Medicine, Division of Emergency Medicine, Harvard Medical School, 75 Francis Street, Boston, Massachusetts 02115-6110*

Preface

Airway management defines the specialty of emergency medicine. It is true that the cardiologist can care for acute pulmonary edema or cardiogenic shock as well as the emergency physician can, but if intubation is required, the cardiologist may well need to call upon the emergency physician to accomplish this crucial resuscitative step. The pulmonologist can care for status asthmaticus or severe respiratory failure in chronic obstructive pulmonary disease as well as the emergency physician can, but if intubation is required, the pulmonologist's expertise may be exceeded, and the assistance of the emergency physician may be vital. Although care of these critically ill patients may require the resources of many different specialties working in concert, it is the emergency physician, and often the emergency physician alone, who can provide definitive resuscitative care to all patients, regardless of their complexity, severity, or presenting condition. And it is often the emergency physician alone who is in the hospital 24 hours each day, 365 days each year, ready to respond immediately to a life-threatening airway crisis. These truths are the genesis of the National Emergency Airway Management Course and of this book, which we dedicate to those front-line providers who do so much for so many.

Writing this book has been a labor of love and of an intensity and commitment that reflect our dedication to this aspect of emergency care. We follow in the steps of the giants of our specialty, those who taught us how to think, how to act, and most importantly, when to act. In that spirit, the book is organized into discrete sections and chapters, both to provide in-depth, detailed discussion of important airway topics and to serve as a quick reference or learning guide. Although the principles of airway management in pediatrics are virtually identical to those in adults, separate pediatric sections emphasize subtle differences and the limitations of some airway techniques in children. Much of the material in this book is original and is presented to provide a foundation upon which future works on airway management can build. We have tried to replicate the thought processes that we must execute successfully in seconds if all is to go well and to present them in a straightforward, intelligent manner. We have created new ways to think of various aspects of airway management and how to remember them. The book will be useful for anyone who provides or wishes to learn about emergency airway management. It is tailored for the medical student, the emergency medicine resident, and the practicing emergency physician, whether in a large, tertiary center or as a lone practitioner in a community Emergency Department.

We are grateful to our colleagues and teachers, and especially those gifted instructors in the National Emergency Airway Management Course, many of whom have contributed to this book. Most of all, we are grateful to our students, whose questions continually push us to think critically and to keep exploring.

Acknowledgments

My life is a wonderful journey, shared by my wife, Barbara, inspired by my students and residents, and made joyous by my children, Andrew, Blake, and Alexa. This book, and all that I do, is really for them. Thanks also to Diane Pugh, whose incredible attention to detail makes everything better than it otherwise would be, and to my faculty at Brigham and Women's Hospital, whose individual and collective search for excellence is a constant source of pride.

RMW

I wish to acknowledge my family, my partners in founding and developing this educational endeavor, the faculty that make it possible to deliver it, and the students who drive us to the cutting edge of emergency airway management.

MFM

To my wife and best friend, Kathleen Ann Rheingans, for her infinite love and support. To my children, Erin Elizabeth, Lauren Banuvar, and Ian Paul Harlan for their honesty and humor which keeps me grounded and humble. To my mentor and close friend, John Andrew Marx, who continuously shows me how one achieves their potential for greatness. Finally, to my fellow editors, Ron, Mike, and Bob with great thanks for their hard work, encouragement and friendship that made this book and the Airway Course a reality.

RES

At this point in my life I have come to realize that any contribution I make has little to do with my own limited ability, but is the product of the influence and gifts of others. I wish to first thank my wife Cindi for her support and for allowing me to have the joys of a family life while still enjoying the privilege of creative work. I would like to acknowledge the students who utilize this information and teach me daily. To my friends Ron, Mike, and Bob who have given me this opportunity and inspire me to do the best I am able to do. And lastly, but most importantly, to my God who is responsible for all of this and has given me the wisdom to understand my role.

RCL

SECTION 1

Approach to the Airway

1

The Decision to Intubate

Ron M. Walls

Chairman, Department of Emergency Medicine, Brigham and Women's Hospital;
Associate Professor of Medicine, Division of Emergency Medicine,
Harvard Medical School, Boston, Massachusetts

Airway management is the single most important skill of the emergency physician. Some say it is the defining skill of emergency medicine. Failure or loss of the airway, with resultant failure of ventilation and oxygenation, is the terminal pathway for many emergency patients. Timely, effective, and decisive management of the airway can quite literally make the difference between life and death or between ability and disability.

Responsibility for definitive management of the airway rests with the emergency physician, who must be capable of utilizing a myriad of airway intervention techniques and, equally important, of deciding when, how, and on whom they should be used. The emergency physician must be proficient with rapid sequence intubation, which requires a thorough knowledge of the pharmacology and effects of neuromuscular blocking agents, sedative or induction agents, and other medications used to improve outcome or mitigate adverse effects. The entire repertoire of airway skills must be mastered, ranging from bag-and-mask ventilation through rapid sequence intubation, awake intubation techniques, steps to be taken in the event of airway difficulty or failure, and, finally, surgical airway techniques. Emergency airway management requires diligent maintenance of a knowledge base, sound clinical judgment, and the decisiveness to act when action is indicated. In many cases, delays in airway decisions create increasing difficulty and magnify the chances of failure and bad outcome.

This chapter focuses on the decision to intubate. Subsequent chapters will describe the technique of rapid sequence intubation and its place in the emergency airway algorithm. Regardless of the actual airway technique that is used, a great proportion of the patient's outcome rests on the initial decision to intubate.

In all cases, the airway itself is paramount and takes precedence over all other clinical considerations. The airway is rightfully allocated the "A" in the ABC of resuscitation. Assessment, establishment, and protection of the airway with assurance of optimal oxygenation and ventilation constitute the foundation on which all other resuscitative measures are based. Without a secure airway and adequate oxygenation and ventilation, all other resuscitative measures are doomed to failure. With the exception of the immediate defibrillation of the cardiac arrest patient, no single resuscitative maneuver takes priority over management of the airway.

I. Indications for intubation

The decision to intubate is based on three fundamental clinical assessments:

1. Is there a failure of airway maintenance or protection?
2. Is there a failure of ventilation or oxygenation?
3. What is the anticipated clinical course?

The results of these three evaluations will lead to a correct decision to intubate or not to intubate in virtually all conceivable cases. Although some would advocate the use of a list of indications for intubation, such lists tend to be difficult to recall in critical situations, and, in any case, can be derived from a fundamental set of principles. These principles are embodied in the three preceding clinical assessments.

A. *Is there a failure of airway maintenance or protection?*

The conscious, alert patient uses the musculature of the upper airway and various protective reflexes to maintain a patent airway and to protect against the aspiration of foreign substances, gastric contents, or secretions. In the severely ill, compromised, or unconscious patient, such airway maintenance and protection mechanisms are often attenuated or lost. A patent airway is essential for adequate oxygenation and ventilation, and protection of this airway against aspiration of gastric contents is vital. If the patient cannot maintain an adequate airway, an artificial airway may be established by inserting an oropharyngeal airway or a nasopharyngeal airway; however, such airway devices do not provide for protection of the airway. In general, any patient who requires the establishment of an airway also requires protection of that airway, and the use of an oropharyngeal or nasopharyngeal airway should be considered a temporizing measure. A patient with a spontaneously patent airway and adequate respiration may be unable to protect the airway against aspiration of gastric contents, which carries a significant morbidity and mortality. It has been taught that assessment of the gag reflex is a reliable method of evaluating protective airway reflexes. In fact, this has never been subjected to adequate scientific scrutiny, and the absence of a gag reflex is neither sensitive nor specific as an indicator of loss of protective airway reflexes. A better clinical assessment is probably afforded by evaluating the ability to swallow spontaneously and to handle secretions. Swallowing is a very complex reflex that requires the patient to sense the presence of material in the oropharynx and then to execute a series of very intricate and coordinated muscular actions to direct the secretions down past a closed airway into the esophagus. Although this concept also has not been adequately studied, the assessment of spontaneous or volitional swallowing is probably a better tool for determining the ability to protect the airway than is the presence or absence of a gag reflex. In the absence of an immediately reversible condition, such as opioid overdose or reversible cardiac dysrhythmia, immediate intubation is indicated for any patient who cannot maintain and protect the airway. A common clinical error occurs when a patient is evaluated and found to be "breathing on his own." Although it may indeed be true that the spontaneous ventilation is adequate, the patient may be at risk for serious aspiration. Some conditions may not threaten the airway immediately, but the natural progress of the disorder will be to encroach further on the airway, eventually causing complete obstruction; therefore early intubation is prudent (see later).

B. *Is there failure of ventilation or oxygenation?*

Oxygenation of the vital organs is the primary function of the respiratory system. Although ventilation and disposal of waste product carbon dioxide are important for pH balance, it is oxygen that is vital for survival. If the patient cannot ventilate adequately or if adequate oxygenation cannot be achieved despite supplemental oxygen, then intubation is indicated. In such cases, the intubation is being performed to facilitate ventilation and oxygenation, rather than simply to establish or protect the airway. An example is the patient with status asthmaticus who will generally maintain and protect the airway even when in extremis. However, ultimately, fatigue will produce ventilatory failure, and resultant hypoxemia will lead to death without intervention. Similarly, the patient with severe pulmonary edema may again be maintaining and protecting the airway but may have progressive oxygenation failure that can only be managed with positive-pressure ventilation through an endotracheal tube. Although some of these patients can be managed with noninvasive ventilatory techniques, such as bilevel continuous positive airway pressure, many still require intubation. Unless ventilatory failure is due to a reversible cause, such as opioid overdose, intubation is mandatory.

C. *What is the expected clinical course?*

Most patients who require intubation in the emergency department have one or more of the previously discussed indications: airway maintenance, airway protection, oxygenation, or ventilation. However, there is another patient for whom intubation is indicated but for whom none of these four fundamental elements is present. This is the patient about whom it can be predicted that his or her currently acceptable anatomy and physiology will deteriorate or for whom the work of breathing will be overwhelming in the face of multiple major injuries. For example, consider the patient who presents with a stab wound to the midzone of the anterior neck and an apparently enlarging hematoma. At the time of presentation, the patient may have perfectly adequate airway maintenance and protection and be ventilating and oxygenating well. However, delay will allow further encroachment on the airway by the hematoma, leading to airway catastrophe and death. Further, the anatomic distortion caused by the enlarged hematoma may well thwart various airway management techniques that would be successful if undertaken earlier. The same consideration applies to the polytrauma patient who presents with hypotension, multiple bilateral rib fractures, a tender abdomen, pelvic fracture, femoral fracture, and mild head injury with combative behavior. Although this patient has adequate airway maintenance and protection, and ventilation and oxygenation may be acceptable, intubation is indicated as part of the management of this constellation of injuries. The reason for the intubation becomes clear when one examines the expected clinical course of this patient. The hypotension mandates aggressive fluid resuscitation and evaluation for the source of the blood loss, including diagnostic peritoneal lavage, abdominal ultrasound, or abdominal computed tomography (CT) scan. Any of these maneuvers will require a significant degree of patient cooperation. The pelvic fracture, if unstable, requires fixation and embolization of bleeding vessels. The femoral fracture will certainly require operative intervention. Chest tubes may be required for one or both hemithoraces to treat hemopneumothorax or in preparation for positive-pressure ventilation during surgery. Finally, the combative behavior pertaining to the head injury may mandate a head CT scan or placement of an intracranial pressure monitor, depending on the other injury priorities. With the patient's ultimate destination certain to include the operating room, and the complex and potentially painful series of procedures and diagnostic evaluations required, this patient is best served by early intubation. In addition, the prolonged hypotension and the body's metabolic response to the injuries will make the work of breathing increasingly challenging for the patient, and ventilatory failure will supervene. Sometimes the clinical course may be uncertain and the patient may be exposed to a period of increased risk. For example, the patient who appears relatively stable with a series of injuries might be appropriate for observation of the airway in the emergency department. If that same patient requires CT scan or angiography or any other prolonged diagnostic procedure, it may be more appropriate to intubate the patient before allowing him or her to leave the department, so that an airway crisis will not ensue in the radiology suite. Similarly, if such a patient were to be transferred from one hospital to another, airway management may be mandated on the basis of the increased risk to the patient during that transfer. This is not to say that every trauma patient or every patient with a serious medical disorder requires intubation;

rather, it is important for the physician to consider the condition in the context of the area in which subsequent care will be provided. If the patient will be leaving the relative safety of the emergency department for a prolonged period of time and the airway is potentially at risk, steps must be taken to ensure that the airway will be preserved and protected and that ventilation and oxygenation will be maintained throughout.

II. Approach to the patient

When the patient presents to the emergency department, the first assessment should be of the patency and adequacy of the airway. In many cases, the adequacy of the airway is confirmed by having the patient speak. Questions such as, "What is your name?" or, "Do you know where you are?" provide both information about the neurologic status and valuable information about the airway. Presence of a normal voice, the ability to inhale and exhale in the modulated manner required for speech, and the ability to comprehend the question and follow instructions provide strong evidence of adequate upper-airway function. Although such an evaluation should not be taken as proof that the upper airway is intact and functioning, it is strongly suggestive that the airway is adequate for the time being. More important, inability of the patient to phonate properly, stridorous sounds from the upper airway, or altered mental status precluding response to the questions would mandate more detailed assessment of the adequacy of airway function and ventilation. Following this introductory evaluation, a more detailed examination of the mouth and oropharynx should be conducted. The mouth should be examined for bleeding; swelling of the tongue or uvula; abnormalities of the oropharynx, such as peritonsillar abscess; or any other abnormalities that might interfere with the free passage of air through the mouth and oropharynx. The mandible and central face should be examined briefly for integrity. Careful examination of the anterior neck requires both visual inspection for deformity, asymmetry, or abnormality, and palpation of the anterior neck, including the larynx and trachea. During palpation, the presence of subcutaneous air should be sought. This is identified by a crackling feeling on compression of the cutaneous tissues of the neck, much as if a sheet of wrinkled tissue paper was lying immediately beneath the skin. When only a small amount of subcutaneous air is present, this physical finding may be subtle and transient and must be sought carefully. Presence of subcutaneous air indicates disruption of an air-filled passage, often the airway itself, especially in the setting of blunt or penetrating chest or neck trauma. Subcutaneous air in the neck can also be caused by esophageal rupture, or rarely, by gas-forming infections. Although these latter two conditions are not immediately threatening to the airway, patients may rapidly deteriorate, requiring subsequent airway management in any case.

After inspection and palpation of the upper airway, the respiratory pattern of the patient should be noted. The presence of respiratory stridor, however slight, indicates some degree of upper-airway obstruction. Stridor is audible without a stethoscope and should not be confused with intermittent expiratory moaning, which is often exhibited by patients in pain. Careful auscultation of the neck with a stethoscope can reveal subclinical stridor that indicates mild airway compromise. Usually, significant airway compromise must develop before any sign of stridor is evident. When evaluating the respiratory pattern, the chest should also be observed. Symmetric, concordant chest movement is the expected finding. In cases where there is significant injury, paradoxical movement of a flail segment of the chest may be observed. If spinal cord injury has disturbed intercostal muscle functioning, diaphragmatic breathing may be present. In this form of breathing, there is little movement of the chest wall and inspiration is evidenced by apparent increase in abdominal volume caused by descent of the diaphragm. Auscultation of the chest will provide clues as to the adequacy of the air exchange. Decreased breath sounds caused by pneumothorax, hemothorax, or other pulmonary pathology are detected.

The assessment of ventilation and oxygenation is a clinical one. Arterial blood gas determination provides little additional information to assess whether intubation is necessary. The clinical impression of the patient's mentation, degree of fatigue, and severity of concomitant injuries or conditions is more important than isolated or a even series of values of P_aO_2 or P_aCO_2. With the advent of pulse oximetry, oxygen saturation can be measured transcutaneously, and arterial blood gases are rarely indicated for the purpose of determining arterial oxygen tensions. In certain circumstances, oxygen saturation monitoring is unsuccessful because of abnormal peripheral perfusion, and arterial blood gases may then be required to assess oxygenation. Measurement of arterial carbon dioxide tension will contribute little useful information to a decision about the need for intubation. In patients with obstructive lung disease, such as asthma or chronic obstructive pulmonary disease, intubation may be required with relatively low carbon dioxide tensions because of patient fatigue. Other times, extremely high carbon dioxide tensions may be managed successfully without intubation. Thus arterial blood gases may add minimal useful information about the need to intubate and may be misleading.

Finally, after assessment of the upper airway and the patient's ventilatory status, including pulse oximetry and mentation, an evaluation of the patient's short-term prognosis is required. If the patient's condition is such that intubation is inevitable and a series of interventions is required, early intubation is preferable. Similarly, if the patient has a condition that is likely to worsen over time and if such worsening is likely to compromise the airway, early airway management is indicated. The same consideration applies to patients who require interhospital transfer by air or ground transportation. Intubation before transfer is vastly preferable to a difficult, uncontrolled intubation during transfer when the condition has worsened. In all circumstances, the decision to intubate should be given precedence. If doubt exists as to whether the patient requires intubation, error should occur on the side of intubating the patient. It is better to intubate the patient, manage the ventilation and the patient for a period of time, and then extubate the patient than to leave the patient without a secure airway and permit an irreversible catastrophe.

ADDITIONAL READING

Benumof JL. Indications for tracheal intubation. In: Benumof JL, ed. *Airway management: principles and practice.* St Louis: Mosby, 1996.

Clinton JE, McGill JW. Basic airway management and decision-making. In: Roberts JR, Hedges JR, eds. *Clinical procedures in emergency medicine,* 3rd ed. Philadelphia: WB Saunders, 1998.

Walls RM. Advanced airway management. In: Rosen P, Barkin R, Danzl DF, et al., eds. *Emergency medicine: concepts and clinical practice,* 4th ed. St Louis: Mosby, 1998.

Walls RM. Airway management. In: Rund DA, Barkin RM, Rosen P, et al., eds. *Essentials of emergency medicine,* 2nd ed. St Louis: Mosby, 1996.

2

Rapid Sequence Intubation

Ron M. Walls

Chairman, Department of Emergency Medicine, Brigham and Women's Hospital;
Associate Professor of Medicine, Division of Emergency Medicine,
Harvard Medical School, Boston, Massachusetts

I. **Definition**

Rapid sequence intubation (RSI) is the administration of a potent induction agent followed immediately by a rapidly acting neuromuscular blocking agent to induce unconsciousness and motor paralysis for tracheal intubation. The technique is predicated on the fact that the patient has not fasted before intubation and is therefore at risk for aspiration of gastric contents. Administration of the drugs is preceded by a preoxygenation phase to permit a period of apnea to occur safely between the administration of the drugs and intubation of the trachea *without interposed assisted ventilation.* In other words, the purpose of RSI is to render the patient unconscious and paralyzed and to then intubate the trachea without the use of bag ventilation, which may cause gastric distention and increase the risk of aspiration. As such, RSI is a clearly defined concept that can be said to consist of a series of discrete steps.

II. **Indications and contraindications**

RSI is the cornerstone of emergency airway management. Other techniques, such as blind nasotracheal intubation or intubation using sedation and topical anesthesia may be useful in patients presenting with a difficult airway. However, the superiority of RSI in terms of success rates, complication rates, and control of adverse effects makes it the procedure of choice for most emergency department intubations. The indications for RSI have been discussed in Chapter 1. There are no absolute contraindications. The cardinal principle in assessing the patient for RSI is the determination of whether the patient is likely to be successfully intubated and, if not, to be successfully ventilated. Difficult intubation per se is not a contraindication to RSI; rather, it indicates to the physician that a careful preintubation plan must be made with a particular emphasis on the ability to ventilate the patient should intubation prove unsuccessful (Chapters 3 and 5). Other relative contraindications pertain more to the choice of individual agents for the intubation than to the use of a rapid sequence technique. These contraindications are discussed in various places throughout this text and within the discussions of the pharmacology of each individual agent.

III. **Description of the technique**

RSI can be thought of as a series of discrete steps, the seven Ps. These are shown in Box 2.1:

A. **Preparation**

Before initiating the sequence, all preparations must be made. The patient must be assessed carefully for the presence of a difficult airway and for the likelihood of success-

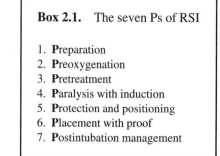

Box 2.1. The seven Ps of RSI

1. **P**reparation
2. **P**reoxygenation
3. **P**retreatment
4. **P**aralysis with induction
5. **P**rotection and positioning
6. **P**lacement with proof
7. **P**ostintubation management

ful bag/mask ventilation, should intubation prove difficult or impossible (Chapters 3 and 5). Fallback plans in the event of failed intubation must be established and the necessary equipment must be close at hand. The patient should be in an area of the emergency department that is organized and equipped for resuscitation. Cardiac monitoring, blood pressure monitoring, and pulse oximetry should be used in all cases. The patient should have at least one secure, well-functioning intravenous line. It is prudent for the physician to assess the patency of this intravenous line personally. It is advisable, when possible, to have a second intravenous line established and running well before initiation of the sequence, in the event the primary intravenous access is compromised. The patient should be positioned on the stretcher and the stretcher should be located in the room so as to optimize the access for intubation (Chapter 6). The sequence of pharmacologic agents should be determined and all agents drawn up in properly labeled syringes. All equipment should be tested. There should be at least two functioning laryngoscope handles and a variety of blades, usually two different sizes each of curved and straight blades. A good, basic set of airway equipment consists of two laryngoscope handles, numbers 3 and 4 MacIntosh laryngoscope blades, and numbers 2 and 3 Miller laryngoscope blades. The blade of choice should be affixed to the laryngoscope handle and clicked into the "On" position to ensure that the light functions and is bright. The light bulbs on each of the laryngoscope blades should be hand-tightened to ensure that they are firmly seated. The endotracheal tube (ETT) size should be chosen based on the patient's anatomy. In general, an 8- or 8.5-mm ETT should be used for adult men and a 7.5- or 8.0-mm tube should be used for adult women. If difficult intubation is anticipated, a smaller tube (6.0 or 6.5 mm) should be prepared as well. Pediatric tube sizes are discussed in Chapter 12. The ETT cuff should be tested by inflation of air and then gentle palpation of the cuff to ensure that there is no air leak. This can be done within the ETT package to maintain sterility without the necessity of wearing sterile gloves. The cuff should then be deflated. A stylet should be used for virtually all intubations. The stylet allows the tube to be formed into a shape that will improve geometric access to the airway. There are two recommended methods of shaping the tube to facilitate intubation. The first is the "hockey stick" method in which the stylet is left completely straight with the exception of the distal 4 or 5 cm, which are bent to form an angle of approximately 45 degrees. The second method is to use the stylet to make a smooth, gentle curve with the entire ETT. The hockey stick configuration may be preferable, as it permits the intubator to direct the distal tip of the tube anteriorly while easily identifying the exact position of the tube because of the straight shaft. When the stylet is placed, care must be taken to ensure that the tip of the stylet does not protrude through the end of the ETT or through the small distal side port (Murphy's eye). After the stylet has been placed, it should be tested to ensure that it can be removed. With the tube configured in the desired manner for intubation, the proximal tip of the ETT is held and the stylet is pulled back to ensure that it can be successfully removed after intubation. After the stylet is appropriately shaped and placed, the proximal end of the stylet should be bent at a sharp angle over the proximal ETT adapter. This will prevent any tendency of the stylet to slide distally in the ETT, possibly leading to protrusion of the tip and damage to the airway. Throughout this preparatory phase, the patient should be receiving preoxygenation, as described later. Care and time taken during this preparation and assessment phase of intubation pay great dividends when the sequence is initiated.

B. Preoxygenation

Preoxygenation is essential to the "no bagging" principle of RSI. Preoxygenation is the establishment of an oxygen reservoir within the lungs and body tissue to permit several minutes of apnea to occur without arterial oxygen desaturation. The principal reservoir is the functional residual capacity in the lungs, which is approximately 30 ml/kg. Administration of 100% oxygen for 5 minutes replaces this predominantly nitrogenous mixture of room air with oxygen, allowing several minutes of apnea time before hemoglobin saturation decreases to less than 90%. Preoxygenation is not simply the establishment of an oxygen reservoir within the lungs; it also involves creating an oxygen surplus in blood and body tissue. A combination of these factors permits prolonged apnea without significant oxygen desaturation. Time to desaturation varies, depending on the patient (Figure 2.1).

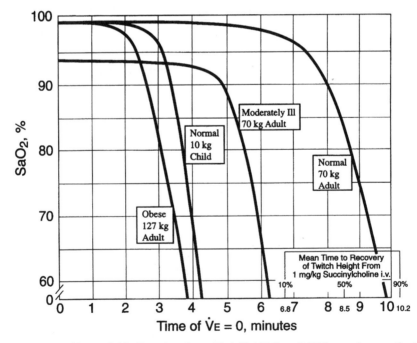

FIG. 2.1. Time to Hemoglobin Desaturation with initial $F_AO_2 = 0.87$ for various patient circumstances. Note the bars indicating recovery from succinylcholine paralysis on the bottom right. Healthy adult patients desaturate to 80% before regaining 50% muscle function after succinylcholine, but virtually all others reach 0 oxygen saturation before recovering even 10% muscle function. (From Benumof J, Dagg R, Benumof R. Critical hemoglobin desaturation will occur before return to an unparalyzed state following 1mg/kg intravenous succinylcholine. *Anesthesiology* 1997;87:979–982, with permission.)

A healthy, fully preoxygenated 70kg adult will maintain oxygen saturation over 90% for 8 minutes, whereas an obese (127 kg) adult will desaturate to 90% in less than 3 minutes. A 10-kg child will desaturate to 90% in less than 4 minutes. The time for desaturation from 90% to 0 is even more important and is much shorter. The healthy 70kg adult desaturates from 90% to 0 in less than 120 seconds, and the small child does so in 45 seconds.

Most emergency departments do not use systems that are capable of delivering 100% oxygen. The most commonly used device is the nonrebreather oxygen mask, which probably delivers oxygen concentrations in the 70% to 75% range. Although, in most cases, preoxygenation using such a device will provide an adequate oxygen reservoir to permit several minutes of apnea without significant desaturation, it is preferable to provide 100% oxygen. A ventilation bag and mask can be placed over the patient's mouth and nose, allowing the patient to breathe the 100% oxygen actively (without assist) from the bag, although this may require the assistance of another person. The use of pulse oximetry throughout intubation enables the physician to monitor the level of oxygen saturation, thus eliminating guesswork. In some circumstances, it is impossible to preoxygenate a patient for 5 minutes before administration of the paralytic drug. In such cases, an equivalent preoxygenation effect can be obtained by having the patient take eight vital-capacity breaths (the largest breaths the patient is capable of taking) in rapid succession (with interposed exhalation) from a 100% oxygen source. This will achieve approximately equivalent nitrogen washout.

C. Pretreatment

Pretreatment is the administration of drugs to mitigate adverse effects associated with the intubation. The administration of 1.5 mg/kg of lidocaine intravenously 3 minutes before intubation mitigates the bronchospastic reactivity of the airways to the ETT in acute severe asthma and blunts the intracranial pressure (ICP) response to intubation in cases of elevated ICP. Other drugs can be used to blunt the sympathetic discharge and ICP increase that accompany laryngoscopy and intubation. There are also circumstances in which it is desirable to administer a small, "defasciculating" dose of a competitive neuromuscular blocking agent 3 minutes before the administration of succinylcholine. These clinical circumstances and the drugs used to affect them are discussed in the various sections throughout this textbook. The drugs themselves can be remembered using the mnemonic "LOAD" as shown in Box 2.2 and in chapter 16.

D. Paralysis with induction

Although this is perhaps the most vital step in the sequence, the likelihood of success will have been greatly increased by the careful assessment, preparation, preoxygenation, and pretreatment that have already occurred. In this phase, a rapidly acting in-

---

Box 2.2.   Pretreatment drugs for RSI

Lidocaine	for reactive airway disease or ↑ICP
Opioid (fentanyl)	when sympathetic responses should be blunted (↑ICP, aortic dissection, ruptured aortic or berry aneurysm, ischemic heart disease)
Atropine	for children ≤ 10 years old
Defasciculation	for ↑ICP

duction agent is given in a dose adequate to produce prompt loss of consciousness. Administration of the induction agent is followed immediately by the neuromuscular blocking agent, usually succinylcholine. Both of these medications are given by intravenous push. The concept of RSI does not involve the slow administration of the induction agent, nor does it involve a titration-to-end-point approach. The sedative agent and dose should be selected with the intention of rapid intravenous administration of the drug. Although rapid administration of these induction agents can increase the likelihood and severity of side effects, especially hypotension, the entire technique is predicated on rapid loss of consciousness, rapid neuromuscular blockade, and a brief period of apnea without interposed assisted ventilation before intubation. Therefore the induction agent is given as a rapid push followed immediately by a rapid push of the succinylcholine. Within a few seconds of the administration of the induction agent and succinylcholine, the patient will begin to lose consciousness and respirations will decrease.

E. Protection and positioning

After 20 to 30 seconds, apnea universally will be present. Sellick's maneuver, the application of firm pressure (about 10 pounds) on the cricoid cartilage to prevent passive regurgitation of gastric contents, should be initiated immediately on the observation that the patient is losing consciousness. If Sellick's maneuver is applied too early, the patient may find it uncomfortable, or vomiting may ensue. Sellick's maneuver should be maintained throughout the entire intubation sequence until the ETT has been correctly placed, the positioned verified, and the cuff inflated. It is often stated that Sellick's maneuver must be discontinued immediately on the initiation of active vomiting by the patient to prevent the possibility of esophageal rupture. This recommendation, although probably correct, has little bearing on the performance of RSI during which the patient is paralyzed, because vomiting requires coordinated neuromuscular activity.

Sellick's maneuver is an essential part of the protection of the airway during RSI and must be performed properly by trained personnel. Also central to protection against aspiration is the avoidance of bag-and-mask ventilation during the intubation sequence. Some patients, as discussed in chapter 22, will be significantly compromised and will require assisted ventilation to maintain oxygen saturations over 90% before, during, and after the intubation. Such patients, especially those with profound hypoxemia, should be bag-and-mask ventilated throughout the sequence to prevent hypoxemia. However, most patients will not require such oxygen supplementation and will be fully protected by a properly conducted preoxygenation phase. If bag-and-mask ventilation is necessary, Sellick's maneuver should be applied to minimize the likelihood of gastric distention and the risk of regurgitation with aspiration. Position the patient for laryngoscopy (Chapter 6).

F. Placement and proof

Approximately 45 seconds after the administration of the succinylcholine, the patient's jaw should be tested for flaccidity and intubation should be undertaken. Because of the *minutes* of safe apnea time permitted by the preoxygenation, the intubation can be performed gently and carefully with due attention to the patient's dentition and proper technique to minimize the potential for trauma to the airway. The glottic aperture should be visualized and the ETT should be placed. The stylet should be removed and the ETT cuff should be inflated. Tube placement should be confirmed as described in Chapter 4 to prove that the tube is correctly placed within the trachea. Sellick's maneuver can then be discontinued on the order of the intubator.

G. Postintubation management

After placement is confirmed, the ET tube must be taped or tied in place. Mechanical ventilation should be initiated as described in Chapter 29. A chest radiograph should be obtained to assess pulmonary status and ensure that mainstream intubation has not occurred. Blood pressure should be measured, and if significant hypotension is present, the management steps in Box 2.3 should be undertaken.

Bradycardia in the postintubation period should always be assumed to be due to esophageal intubation with hypoxia until this is absolutely disproven. Hypertension in the postintubation period usually indicates inadequate sedation. Long-term sedation and paralysis should be administered using a benzodiazepine (e.g., diazepam 0.2 mg/kg) and a competitive neuromuscular blocking agent (e.g., pancuronium 0.1 mg/kg or vecuronium 0.1 mg/kg). An opioid analgesic, such as morphine 0.1 to 0.2 mg/kg, may be added to improve patient comfort. The benzodiazepine and opioid should be repeated in approximately one-third of the initial dose when any signs of patient awareness are detected (especially tachycardia or hypertension), or not less frequently than hourly until it is desirable to allow the patient to recover consciousness. The neuromuscular blocking agent should be repeated as a dose of one-third the original dose (generally, 2 to 3 mg in an adult patient) every 45 to 60 minutes, or when any motor activity is detected.

IV. Timing the steps of rapid sequence intubation

Successful RSI requires a detailed knowledge not only of the precise steps to be taken but also of the time required for each step to achieve its purpose. Preoxygenation requires 5 minutes for maximal effect. In hurried circumstances, especially with ongoing oxygen saturation monitoring, eight vital-capacity breaths can accomplish approximately the same preoxygenation effect in less than 30 seconds. It is recommended that pretreatment drugs be given 3 minutes before the administration of the sedative and neuromuscular blocking agent. The pharmacokinetics of the sedatives and neuromuscular blockers would indicate that a 45-second interval between administration of these agents and initiation of endotracheal intubation is optimal. Thus the entire sequence of RSI can be described as a series of timed steps. For the purposes of discussion, time zero is the time at which the succinylcholine is pushed. The recommended sequence is shown Box 2.4.

Box 2.3. Hypotension in the postintubation period

Cause	Detection	Action
Tension pneumothorax	Increased peak inspiratory pressure (PIP), difficulty bagging, decreased breath sounds, poor O_2 saturation	Immediate thoracostomy
Decreased venous return	Usually seen in patients with high PIPs secondary to high intrathoracic pressure	Fluid bolus, treatment of airway resistance (bronchodilators); increase expiratory time; try $\downarrow V_T$
Induction agents	Other causes excluded	Fluid bolus, expectant
Cardiogenic	Usually in compromised patient; ECG; exclude other causes	Fluid bolus (caution) pressors

---

Box 2.4.   The sequence of RSI

Time	Action (seven Ps)
Zero minus 10 minutes	**P**reparation: *Assemble all necessary equipment, drugs, etc.*
Zero minus 5 minutes	**P**reoxygenation
Zero minus 3 minutes	**P**retreatment
Zero	**P**aralysis with induction: *Administer induction agent by IV push, followed immediately by paralytic agent by IV push*
Zero plus 20 to 30 seconds	**P**rotection: *Apply Sellick's maneuver; position patient for optimal laryngoscopy*
Zero plus 45 seconds	**P**lacement: *Assess mandible for flaccidity, perform intubation; Confirm Placement*
Zero plus 1 minute	**P**ostintubation management: *See text for details*

V. Success rates and complications

Rapid sequence intubation has a success rate approaching 100% in the emergency department. Reported success rates have been very high and exceed those of any other technique. The National Emergency Airway Registry shows an overall success rate of 99% for RSI in more than 4,000 patients. Principal complications of RSI are the mechanical complications of intubation itself. The most catastrophic complication is unrecognized esophageal intubation. This underscores the importance of the confirmation of tube placement described in Chapter 4. It is incumbent on the person who administers neuromuscular blocking agents and potent sedatives to the patient to be able to establish an airway and maintain mechanical ventilation. This may require a surgical airway as a final rescue for a failed oral intubation attempt (Chapters 3, 5, 9, and 11). Aspiration of gastric contents can occur but is uncommon. Alterations in heart rate and blood pressure can result from the pharmacologic agents used or from stimulation of the larynx with resultant reflexes. Specific complications can arise with the use of virtually all the induction agents. These are described in Chapter 15. Overall, the true complication rate of RSI in the emergency department is low and the success rate is exceedingly high, especially when one considers the serious nature of the illnesses for which patients are intubated and the limited time and information available to the clinician performing the intubation.

VI. Accelerated and immediate RSI

When time is of the essence, the RSI sequence can be compressed, so that the steps are conducted much more rapidly than the standard RSI outlined earlier.

1. Accelerated RSI

    More rapid intubation can be achieved by:
    - Shortening preoxygenation to 30 seconds by using the eight-vital-capacity-breath method
    - Shortening pretreatment interval to 2 minutes from 3 minutes

2. Immediate RSI
    - Eliminate pretreatment
    - Preoxygenate with eight vital-capacity breaths

VII. Tips and pearls

As with many technical procedures, preparation is the key to success. A little extra time spent in evaluating the patient and planning an appropriate technique will enhance the chances for success. If the airway appears to be potentially extremely difficult, an awake technique may be used to evaluate access to the glottis before giving neuromuscular blocking agents and induction agents (Chapter 8). Always position the patient optimally before attempting intubation (Chapter 6). If the laryngoscopy is not successful at first, take a moment to determine why the glottis cannot be visualized. A straight blade may be required if the epiglottis is long, floppy, or simply in the way. The person performing Sellick's maneuver may have pushed the airway out of the midline, thus obscuring land-marks. Displacement of the larynx backward, upward, and rightward (BURP—backward, upward, rightward pressure) may improve laryngoscopic view. Repositioning of the head and neck may facilitate visualization of the airway. The most important tip for success is to realize that the technique that has been used, including preoxygenation, usually allows *minutes* of laryngoscopy time. Great time and care can be taken because the technique used has optimized the opportunity for success. Oxygen saturation must be monitored continuously and ventilation initiated if the oxygen saturation falls below 90%. If ade-quate visualization is not achieved, the patient should be ventilated with a bag and mask and repositioned, and another attempt at laryngoscopy should be made, making every ef-fort to optimize both patient positioning and the technique. Again, the importance of ver-ification of ETT placement cannot be overstated. Postintubation bradycardia is caused by esophageal intubation until absolutely and reliably proven otherwise.

ADDITIONAL READING

Murphy MF. Elevated intercranial pressure. In: Dailey R, ed. *The airway: emergency management.* St Louis: Mosby, 1992.

Walls RM. Airway management. In: Marx JA, ed. Advances in trauma. *Emerg Med Clin North Am* 1993;11:53–60.

Walls RM. Airway management. In: Rosen P, Barkin R, Danzl DF, et al., eds. *Emergency medicine: concepts and clin-ical practice,* 4th ed. St Louis: Mosby, 1998.

Walls RM. Airway management. In: Rund DA, Barkin RM, Rosen P, et al., eds. *Essentials of emergency medicine,* 2nd ed. St Louis: Mosby, 1996.

Walls RM. The multiple trauma patient. In: Dailey R, ed. *The airway: emergency management.* St Louis: Mosby, 1992:243–258.

Walls RM. Rapid sequence intubation in head trauma. *Ann Emerg Med* 1993;22:1008–1013.

Walls RM, Vissers RJ, Sagarin MJ, et al. 1288 emergency department intubations: final report of the National Emer-gency Airway Registry Pilot Project. Society for Academic Emergency Medicine, *Acad Emerg Med* 1998;5:393(abst).

3

The Emergency Airway Algorithms

Ron M. Walls

*Chairman, Department of Emergency Medicine, Brigham and Women's Hospital;
Associate Professor of Medicine, Division of Emergency Medicine,
Harvard Medical School, Boston, Massachusetts*

Attempts to define a unified approach to airway management have met with mixed success. The American College of Surgeons' Committee on Trauma developed an algorithmic approach to airway management for trauma patients for the Advanced Trauma Life Support Course. Although fundamentally sound, this algorithm is not applicable to patients with medical disorders requiring intubation, and the role of neuromuscular blockade in airway management is inadequately addressed. This chapter discusses the emergency airway algorithms, which consist of a fundamental approach, supplemented by specialized algorithms for the "crash" situation, the difficult airway, and the failed airway. These algorithms are shown in Figures 3.2 to 3.5 and the reader may wish to refer to the figures while reading the following text descriptions. The algorithm does not attempt to define the need for intubation and does not deal with the decision to intubate. These are covered in Chapter 1. Therefore the entry point for the emergency airway algorithm is immediately after the decision to intubate has been made.

A brief overview algorithm has been developed and defines the basic approach to the emergency airway (Figure 3.1). The approach is as follows: When a patient requires intubation, the first evaluation regards whether the patient represents a "crash" scenario (unconscious, near death, agonal or no respirations, expected to be unresponsive to laryngoscopy). If so, the patient is managed as a crash airway (Figure 3.3). If not, the next determination regards whether the patient represents a difficult airway (Chapter 5). If so, the patient is managed as having a difficult airway (Figure 3.4). If neither a crash airway nor a difficult airway is present, then rapid sequence intubation (RSI) is recommended. Regardless of the algorithm used initially (main, crash, or difficult), if airway failure occurs, the failed-airway algorithm is immediately invoked. This is explained in much more detail in the following sections.

I. The main emergency airway management algorithm ("main" algorithm)

The algorithm is shown in Figure 3.2. It begins after the decision to intubate and ends with postintubation management, which may be reached directly or via one of the other algorithms, depending on patient circumstances.

A. Step M-1: Needs intubation

This indicates the starting point of the algorithm. If the patient does not require intubation or if the decision to intubate has not been made, the algorithm should not be entered.

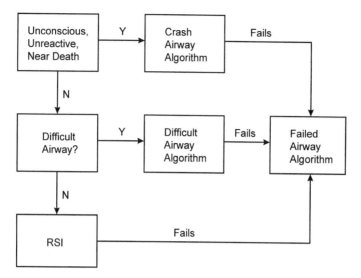

FIG. 3.1. The universal emergency airway algorithm. (See the text for details.)

B. **Step M-2: Is the patient agonal or completely unresponsive?**
The first question that must be asked is, "Is this a crash airway situation?" Indications of a "crash" airway situation include the following:
- Unresponsive patient
- Apnea or agonal respirations
- Arrested or near death
- Anticipated to be unresponsive to laryngoscopy

If these conditions are present, then branch to the crash airway algorithm, shown in Figure 3.3. If the patient is not agonal or shows any response to stimulation, including response to insertion of a laryngoscope, then proceed down the main algorithm to Step M-3.

C. **Step M-2.1: Crash airway**
This represents the exit point from the emergency airway algorithm to the crash algorithm. The next step would be to enter the crash algorithm via Step C-1 in Figure 3.3.

D. **Step M-3: Is the airway predicted to be difficult?**
The assessment of the patient for potentially difficult intubation is described in Chapter 5. It is understood that virtually all emergency intubations are difficult to some extent. However, the evaluation of the patient for attributes that will predict failure of intubation is extremely important. If the patient represents a particularly difficult airway situation, then proceed to the difficult airway algorithm shown in Figure 3.4. If the airway is not felt to be unusually difficult, then proceed down the main algorithm to Step M-4.

E. **Step M-3.1: Difficult airway**
This represents the exit point from the main algorithm and corresponds to the entry point for the difficult airway algorithm via Step D-1 in Figure 3.4.

F. **Step M-4: Rapid sequence intubation**
RSI is the method of choice for airway management in the emergency department. In the absence of a predicted difficult airway or of a "crash" situation as defined earlier, the decision pathway leads to RSI. Rapid sequence intubation is described in detail in

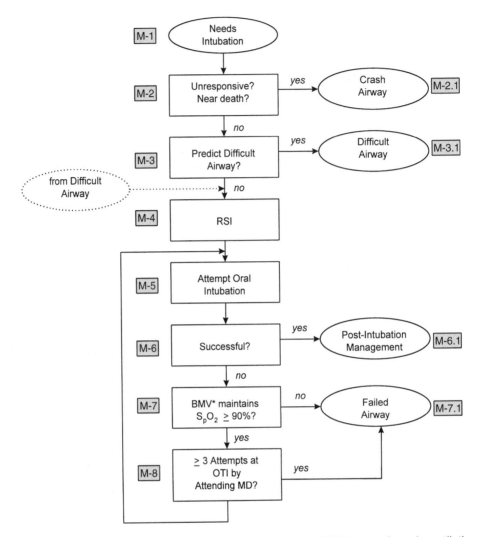

FIG. 3.2. Main emergency airway management algorithm. *BMV, bag-and-mask ventilation.

Chapter 2. RSI affords the best opportunity for success with the least opportunity for adverse outcome of any possible airway method, when applied to appropriately selected patients. This step assumes that the appropriate sequence of preparation, preoxygenation, pretreatment, paralysis with induction, and protection will be followed in preparation for the intubation attempt that will occur in Step M-5. When the patient is in extreme respiratory distress or when haste is required, an accelerated or immediate RSI protocol can be used (Chapter 2).

G. Step M-5: Attempt oral intubation

This is the intubation attempt that occurs as part of the RSI. *An attempt is defined as activities occurring during a single continuous laryngoscopy maneuver.* In other words, if several attempts are made to place an endotracheal tube (ETT) during the course of a single laryngoscopy, this would count as one attempt. This is important because of the definition of airway failure that will come in Step M-8.

H. Step M-6: Is the intubation successful?

If the oral intubation that is attempted in Step M-5 is successful, then branch to post-intubation management via Step M-6.1. If the intubation attempt was not successful, continue on the main pathway.

I. Step M-6.1: Postintubation management

Postintubation management consists of confirmation of ETT placement; use of chest radiography to ascertain the position of the ETT within the trachea; initiation of long-term paralysis and sedation, if desired; and management of the patient's presenting condition. These steps are described in Chapter 2 and throughout this text as part of the discussion of the special clinical circumstances (Chapters 17 to 27).

J. Step M-7: Is bag-and-mask ventilation (BMV) successful?

When the first attempt at intubation is unsuccessful, the appropriate first maneuver is BMV of the patient. This underscores the importance of assessing the likelihood of successful BMV before beginning the intubation sequence. In the vast majority of cases, especially when neuromuscular blockade has been used, BMV will provide adequate ventilation and oxygenation for the patient, defined as maintenance of the oxygen saturation at 90% or higher. If BMV fails, either because of mechanical factors, such as a poor mask seal; anatomic factors, such as massive obesity or pregnancy; impeding chest expansion; or other factors, such as severe pulmonary disease resulting in a failure to achieve adequate oxygenation, then the airway must immediately be defined as failed and management proceeds according to Step M-7.1 to the failed-airway algorithm shown in Figure 3.5. This represents the "can't intubate, can't oxygenate" scenario (Chapter 5).

K. Step M-7.1: Failed airway

To reiterate: The failure of a single attempt at oral intubation followed by a failure to maintain $S_pO_2 \geq 90\%$ with bag and mask constitutes a failed airway and immediate steps should be taken to address it according to the guidelines in Figure 3.5 and the principles in Chapter 5. Enter figure 3.5 at Step F-1.

L. Step M-8: Have three or more attempts at orotracheal intubation been made by an experienced attending physician?

If three separate attempts at orotracheal intubation by direct laryngoscopy by an experienced operator have been unsuccessful, then the airway again is defined as failed despite the ability to bag-ventilate the patient. If three attempts by an experienced operator are unsuccessful, the likelihood of success in the face of further attempts is very small. Therefore the decision should be made to treat the airway as failed and steps should be initiated as described in Figure 3.5 and discussed in Chapter 5.

If this point in the algorithm is reached after a single unsuccessful laryngoscopy or after two unsuccessful attempts at orotracheal intubation but bag ventilation has been successful, then it is appropriate to attempt orotracheal intubation again after a brief period of BMV to ensure adequate oxygenation of the patient. Similarly, if the initial attempts were made by an inexperienced operator, such as a trainee, and the patient is adequately ventilated and oxygenated between attempts, then it is appropriate to reattempt oral intubation until three attempts by an experienced attending physician have been unsuccessful. Thus if less than three attempts have been made, branch back to Step M-5 and again attempt oral intubation. There will be circumstances in which it is clear to an experienced operator that intubation will not be possible after only a single attempt at laryngoscopy. In such cases, if the patient has been optimally placed in the sniffing position; good relaxation has been achieved; the maneuver of backward, upward, rightward, pressure (BURP) has been used; and the operator is convinced that further attempts at laryngoscopy would be futile, the airway should be immediately regarded as failed and appropriate steps should be taken.

II. The crash airway algorithm

A. Step C-1: Crash airway

This is the entry point for the crash algorithm (Figure 3.3), which may be reached via the main algorithm (Figure 3.2, Step M-2.1). Entry at this point connotes an unconscious, unresponsive patient with immediate need for airway management.

B. Step C-2: Attempt oral intubation

The first step in the crash algorithm is to attempt oral intubation immediately by direct laryngoscopy without pharmacologic assist.

C. Step C-3: Is the oral intubation successful?

If yes, then proceed to postintubation management via Step C-3.1, as previously described in the discussion of the main algorithm (Step M-6.1).

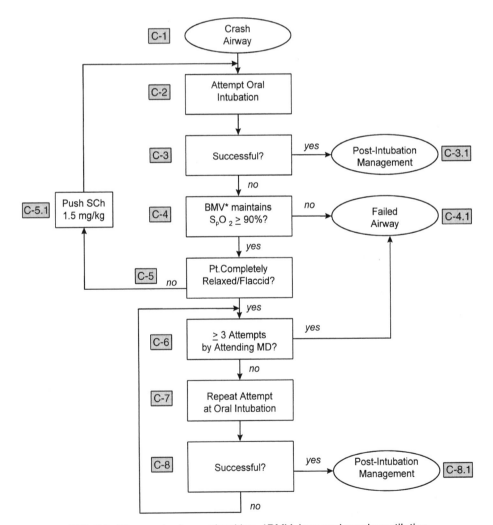

FIG. 3.3. The crash airway algorithm. *BMV, bag-and-mask ventilation

D. Step C-4: Is BMV successful?

If bag ventilation is successful, then further attempts at oral intubation are possible. If BMV is unsuccessful in the context of a failed oral intubation with a crash airway, then a failed airway is present. One further attempt at intubation may be indicated, but no more than one, because intubation has failed and the failure of bag ventilation places the patient in serious and immediate jeopardy. This is a "can't intubate, can't oxygenate" scenario, and in such circumstances, the failed-airway algorithm (Figure 3.5) mandates surgical airway management. If surgical airway management is not *immediately* possible, temporizing methods, such as placement of the intubating laryngeal mask airway (I-LMA) or Combitube, may be attempted, but such attempts should not delay creation of a surgical airway.

E. Step C-4.1: Failed airway (See Figure 3.5).

F. Step C-5: Is the patient completely relaxed and flaccid?

During the first attempt at orotracheal intubation of the unconscious, unresponsive patient, the patient is assessed for the degree of relaxation to permit intubation. If the impression is one of absolute, complete skeletal muscle relaxation, then further intubation attempts are indicated. If the patient is felt to be exhibiting any resistance whatsoever to intubation, then a single dose of succinylcholine 1.5 mg/kg should be given and oral intubation attempted again.

G. Step C-5.1: Succinylcholine 1.5 mg/kg

Succinylcholine is given to ensure complete relaxation of the patient for intubation. Usually, only one dose is indicated. No induction agent is required.

H. Step C-6: Have there been three or more attempts at intubation by an experienced, attending physician?

If the answer to this question is yes, then consistent with the preceding definition, the situation represents a failed airway (Figure 3.5). If fewer than three attempts have been made by an experienced attending physician, then repeated attempts at oral intubation are justified. Between each intubation attempt, defined by a single laryngoscopy, the patient should receive ventilation and oxygenation through a bag and mask.

I. Step C-7: Repeat attempt at oral intubation

It is appropriate to repeat attempts at oral intubation until three attempts have failed. The failure of three attempts indicates a very low likelihood of ultimate success with oral intubation.

J. Step C-8: Successful?

If intubation is achieved, then proceed to postintubation management; if not, cycle back to Step C-6 to make another attempt or to proceed to the failed-airway algorithm, depending on the number of attempts that have already been made.

K. Step C-8.1: Postintubation management

This is undertaken in the event of a successful intubation.

III. The difficult airway

Assessment and management of the difficult airway are discussed in detail in Chapter 5. This algorithm represents the clinical approach that should be used in the event of a perceived difficult airway (Figure 3.4).

A. Step D-1: Difficult airway predicted

The clinician has assessed the patient and determined that the trachea is likely to be unusually difficult to intubate. The "call for assistance" box is represented as a dotted line because this is a purely optional step, dependent on the clinical circumstances, the skill of the physician, available resources, and availability of additional personnel. In circumstances where two emergency physicians are on duty, it may be advisable to inform the

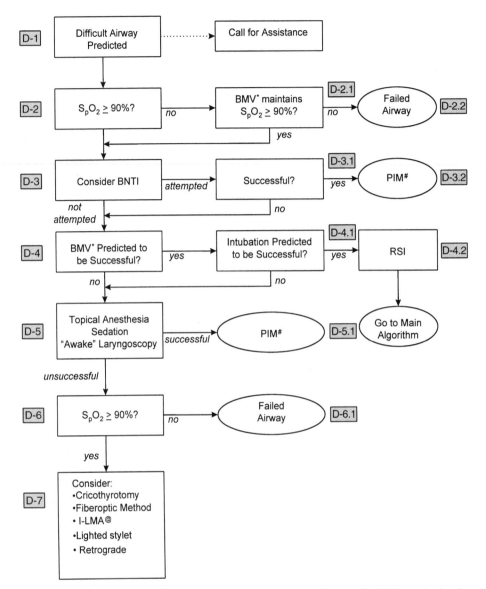

FIG. 3.4. Difficult airway algorithm. *BMV, bag-and-mask ventilation; @I-LMA, intubating laryngeal mask airway (FASTRACH®); #PIM, postintubation management.

second emergency physician of the intubation so that help might be readily available, if required. "Assistance" might include personnel, special airway equipment, or both.

B. Step D-2: Are ventilation and oxygenation adequate?

If ventilation and oxygenation are adequate and oxygen saturation is more than 90%, then a careful assessment and a methodical, planned approach can be undertaken, even if significant preparation time is required. However, if ventilation and oxygenation are inadequate, then immediate steps are required to determine whether adequate ventilation and oxygenation can be achieved by the administration of supplemental oxygenation, BMV, or both.

C. Step D-2.1: Is bag ventilation adequate?

Supplemental oxygen and bag-assisted ventilation may provide adequate oxygenation and ventilation to allow a more methodical and planned approach to the difficult airway. If so, return to the main path down the algorithm. If not, exit via Step D-2.2 to the failed-airway algorithm.

D. Step D-3: Is the patient a candidate for blind nasotracheal intubation?

Arrival at this point in the algorithm implies the patient has adequate oxygenation and ventilation, either spontaneously or with the assistance of a bag and mask. Although the intubation has been determined to be difficult, if the upper airway, including nares and oropharynx, is clear and accessible, and if there is no contraindication to blind nasotracheal intubation (BNTI), then BNTI may be attempted (Chapter 8). The primary indication for BNTI is a need for intubation in a patient who has limited or impossible oral access but in whom the naso- and oropharynx are deemed to be clear and there is no hypopharyngeal pathology in the airway. An example would be a patient with angiotensin-converting enzyme inhibitor–induced angioedema in which the predominant swelling may be in the anterior portion of the tongue and lips. In such patients, the ETT may be passed successfully through the nare and into the trachea via the naso- and oropharynx.

E. Step D-3.1: Attempted/successful?

If blind nasotracheal intubation is attempted and is successful, then proceed to postintubation management via Step D-3.2. If BNTI was either not attempted or unsuccessful, then we return to the main pathway to Step D-4.

F. Step D-4: Is BMV predicted to be successful?

We have now arrived at the point where we have a patient who has adequate oxygenation and ventilation and for whom BNTI either is not useful or has failed. The next step is to consider RSI. This decision hinges on two key questions. The one represented at this point in the algorithm is whether BMV is predicted to be successful. This may already be known if BMV was required at the earlier decision point in Step D-2.1. If the patient has been breathing spontaneously and oxygenating adequately to this point, BMV may have not been attempted. It is necessary to make an assessment about whether BMV is likely to be successful, as this is a virtual prerequisite for RSI. This requires physical assessment and may include a trial of bag-assisted ventilation (Chapter 5).

G. Step D-4.1: Is intubation predicted to be successful?

If BMV is predicted to be successful and there is a reasonable likelihood of success with oral intubation, *despite the difficult airway,* then RSI may be undertaken. If BMV is unlikely to succeed in the context of difficult intubation or if the chance of successful oral intubation is felt to be remote, then RSI is not recommended.

H. Step D-4.2: Consider RSI

See the discussion for Step D-4.1. If RSI is undertaken, enter the main algorithm via the dotted-line box that says, "From Difficult Airway." A double set-up may be desirable.

I. Step D-5: Topical anesthesia and sedation with awake laryngoscopy

At this point in the algorithm, we have a patient who has a predicted difficult airway but who is exhibiting adequate oxygenation and ventilation either spontaneously or with bag-and-mask assist. Blind nasotracheal intubation either is considered inappropriate or has failed, and RSI is believed to be inappropriate because of predicted extreme difficulty with intubation or a combination of difficult intubation and probably unsuccessful BMV. For such patients, the recommended approach is one of awake laryngoscopy. This technique is used either to intubate the patient or to prove that laryngoscopy will result in visualization of the vocal cords, thus permitting RSI. This is described in detail in Chapter 8. Laryngoscopy may be conventional or fiberoptic.

J. Step D-5.1: Postintubation management

If the awake laryngoscopy results in successful intubation or demonstrates that oral intubation will be successful, thus permitting RSI, then move to postintubation management. If awake laryngoscopy is unsuccessful in achieving intubation visualizing the glottis, then further techniques will be required.

K. Step D-6: Ventilation and oxygenation remain adequate?

If at any point during the algorithm, there is a failure of ventilation and oxygenation, defined as inability to maintain $S_pO_2 \geq 90\%$, the situation reverts to that of a failed airway and transfers via Step D-6.1 to the failed-airway algorithm. If ventilation and oxygenation remain adequate, then there are alternative techniques to achieve a functional airway in the difficult airway case.

L. Step D-7:

Consider the following techniques:

- Cricothyrotomy
- Fiberoptic method
- Intubating LMA (I-LMA)
- Lighted stylet
- Retrograde intubation

These techniques are useful in the management of the difficult airway and are described in Chapters 9, 10, and 11. Fiberoptic methods include flexible fiberoptic bronchoscopy with intubation, the Bullard laryngoscope, and other fiberoptic instruments. In any case, if the ability to maintain adequate oxygenation and ventilation is lost, immediate reversion to the failed-airway algorithm is indicated.

IV. The failed airway

At several points in the preceding algorithms, it may be determined that airway management has failed. The definitions of this are outlined earlier in this chapter and in Chapter 5. When a failed airway has been determined to occur, the circumstances are somewhat different, depending on whether BMV is possible and adequate. A recommended approach to the failed airway is described in the following discussion and is shown in Figure 3.5.

A. Step F-1: Failed-airway criteria have been met

This is the entry point of the failed-airway algorithm. The criteria are either three failed attempts at intubation via oral laryngoscopy by an experienced attending physician or a single failed attempt at oral intubation with inability to maintain $S_pO_2 \geq 90\%$ using a bag and mask. A mandated intubation in a patient with a difficult or crash airway in whom BMV fails also represents a failed airway. As with the difficult airway, it may be advisable to call for assistance when a failed airway has occurred. This is especially true if BMV has also failed and if there is qualified help *immediately* available. The assistance may be additional nursing personnel, respiratory therapists, other personnel, equipment, emergency physicians, anesthesiologists, or surgeons.

B. Step F-2: Is BMV possible and adequate?

In the circumstance of a failed airway, if BMV is not adequate, then immediate cricothyrotomy is mandatory. Further attempts at intubation or use of alternate devices will merely prolong the patient's hypoxemic state. The only exception to this recommendation is the use of a temporizing technique, such as TTJV, the I-LMA or Combitube, when cricothyrotomy is not immediately possible. If surgical airway management is itself contraindicated, then alternative methods may be tried first. For example, if the

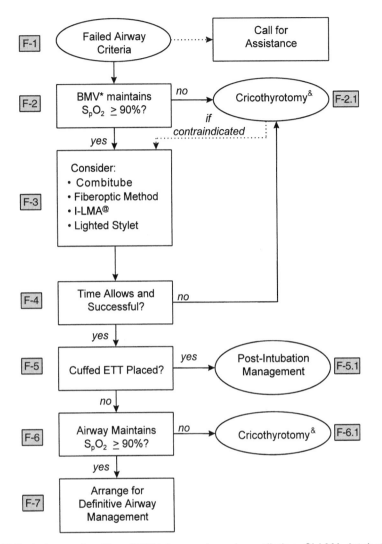

FIG. 3.5. Failed-airway algorithm. *BMV, bag-and-mask ventilation; @I-LMA, intubating laryngeal mask airway; &TTJV, transtracheal jet ventilation, may be used to temporize.

patient has known laryngeal pathology, such as a tumor or hematoma, then alternative techniques may be preferred. However, if these methods are not successful, cricothyrotomy should be performed, even in the presence of contraindications.

C. Step F-2.1: Cricothyrotomy (see the preceding discussion)

D. Step F-3: Consider Combitube, fiberoptic method, I-LMA, or lighted stylet

If ventilation and oxygenation by bag and mask can maintain $S_pO_2 \geq 90\%$, then a number of different devices and procedures may be attempted to rescue the failed airway. At all times, the patient must be monitored for adequate oxygenation. If oxygenation becomes inadequate at any time and cannot be restored via BMV, then cricothyrotomy is mandatory. Likewise, if there is failure of each of the techniques considered appropriate, then cricothyrotomy should be undertaken. Fiberoptic methods include flexible fiberoptic bronchoscopy with intubation, the Bullard laryngoscope, and other fiberoptic devices.

E. Step F-4: Time allows and successful?

See the discussion in Step F-3. If there is sufficient time to achieve oxygenation and ventilation using one of these devices or techniques, then proceed down the main path of the algorithm. If not, cricothyrotomy is mandated.

F. Step F-5: Was cuffed ETT placed?

If the technique that was successful was the placement of an ETT using the lighted stylet, I-LMA, or a fiberoptic method, then a definitive airway has been placed, and postintubation management may be undertaken. If the Combitube or percutaneous transtracheal ventilation has been used, then the airway should be considered temporary at best.

G. Step F-5.1: Postintubation management

H. Step F-6: Airway as placed adequate to ventilate?

If adequate ventilation and oxygenation are achieved by the airway that has been placed, then arrangements must be initiated for definitive airway management, possibly in the operating room. If the airway as placed is inadequate and there is a failure of oxygenation, then cricothyrotomy is indicated.

I. Step F-6.1: Cricothyrotomy

J. Step F-7: Arrange for definitive airway management

See the discussion in Step F-6.

V. Conclusions

The algorithms presented in this chapter represent a recommended approach to airway management in the emergency department. They are intended as guidelines only. Individual decision making, clinical circumstances, skill of the physician, and available resources will determine the final, best approach to airway management in any individual case. Understanding the fundamental concepts of the difficult and failed airway, recognition of the crash circumstances that mandate immediate airway management, and use of RSI as the airway management method of choice for most emergency department patients, however, will result in successful airway management with minimal morbidity in the vast majority of circumstances.

ADDITIONAL READING

American Society of Anesthesiologists Task Force on the Difficult Airway: ASH difficult airway algorithm. *Anesthesiology* 1993;58:597.

Benumof JL. *Airway Management: principles and practice.* St. Louis, MO: Mosby, 1996.

Walls RM. Airway management. In: Rosen P, Barkin R, Danzl DF, et al., eds. *Emergency medicine: concepts and clinical practice,* 4th ed. St Louis: Mosby, 1998.

4

Confirmation of Endotracheal
Tube Placement

Ron M. Walls

*Chairman, Department of Emergency Medicine, Brigham and Women's Hospital,
Associate Professor of Medicine, Division of Emergency Medicine,
Harvard Medical School, Boston, Massachusetts*

Inadvertent intubation of the esophagus can occur during any intubation, despite appropriate and careful technique. This is especially true in the emergency department, where both time and information are limited. There are two important steps in confirmation of appropriate endotracheal tube (ETT) placement:

1. confirmation of tracheal intubation *and*
2. assessment of the position of the ETT within the trachea

I. Confirmation of tracheal intubation

Historically, it has been taught that a combination of clinical evaluations can confirm tracheal intubation. These clinical evaluations have included observation of the ETT passing through the cords during intubation, auscultation of clear and equal bilateral breath sounds, absence on auscultation of air sounds over the epigastrium, observation of symmetric rising and falling of the chest during ventilation, and observation of condensation within the ETT concordant with the ventilatory cycle. Unfortunately, these observations, individually and collectively, are subject to failure and cannot be relied on. Placement of the ETT within the esophagus is an accepted complication of intubation, but failure to recognize and correct it immediately is not. Chest radiography can be used to assess ETT position, but it does not confirm tracheal placement because the esophagus lies immediately behind the trachea, and an ETT placed within the esophagus can appear to be within the trachea on an anterior-posterior (AP) chest x-ray. Lateral chest radiographs are virtually never taken for confirmation of tube placement and take too long to obtain, develop, and view to be useful for tube placement confirmation. Fortunately, three additional devices are now readily available and can help to remove any uncertainty about the placement of the ETT.

A. Pulse oximetry

As described previously, pulse oximetry should be used throughout all emergency department intubations. It has been argued that the use of pulse oximetry precludes the need for any other means of verification of ETT placement because esophageal placement will invariably be accompanied by subsequent oxygen desaturation. Although this is true, proper preoxygenation techniques can delay the onset of such desaturation for several minutes following intubation, thus misleading the caregivers. The desaturation may occur when personnel are somewhat less vigilant than they were immediately following intubation. Desaturation will also occur precipitously, as the oxygen stores have been used and the partial pressure of oxygen has reached the steep part of the oxyhemoglobin dissociation curve (Chapter 2). Also, pulse oximetry may be unreliable because of the patient's clinical status (especially hypotension). Thus when oxygen desaturation is observed, there may be precious little time left for remedy. Therefore although pulse oximetry should be used throughout every intubation, it is not a preferred method of ensuring ETT placement and may even be misleading for a short time.

B. End-tidal CO_2 monitoring

During the ventilatory cycle, the exchange of CO_2 within the alveoli leads to a normal and predictable amount of CO_2 in the exhaled air. Detection of this CO_2 confirms placement of the ETT within the trachea, for esophageal placement will never cause exhalation of gases with sufficient quantities of CO_2, even if the stomach is ventilated for a brief period. Presence of a carbonated beverage in the stomach similarly does not lead to CO_2 production that is capable of "fooling" the end-tidal CO_2 detector. Three primary techniques are used in devices monitoring end-tidal CO_2 for confirmation of ETT placement:

1. colorimetric,
2. qualitative, *and*
3. quantitative

1. Colorimetric end-tidal CO_2 detection

Colorimetric end-tidal CO_2 detection involves the use of a device that is placed between the bag and the ETT. The device is small, disposable, and contains a color indicator that changes according to the concentration of CO_2 in the exhaled air. Typically, the colorimetric indicator changes from purple to yellow on detection of CO_2. When such a color change occurs, the detector is virtually 100% specific for confirmation of tracheal placement of the ETT. Rarely, the tube may be positioned above the glottis, giving rise to a false-positive detection of CO_2. If the tube is within the esophagus, no color change will occur. There is an intermediate zone of color change, usually represented by a tan color. Such a reading should be considered indeterminate and should not be considered to indicate tracheal intubation. In the presence of cardiac arrest, in a small number of cases there may be no color change of the indicator even though the tube is correctly placed within the trachea. This is caused by the profound cessation of CO_2 production and delivery to the lungs for gas exchange. In addition to confounding attempts to confirm ETT placement, such profound and prolonged states of circulatory arrest generally portend an abysmal prognosis. In such cases and where intermediate color change has occurred, repeat laryngoscopy and use of an alternate technique, such as an aspiration device, may be helpful. There is a misconception that the asthmatic patient can have such severe bronchoconstriction that gas exchange will not occur, despite tracheal placement of the tube. This is not true, and absence of CO_2 detection is evidence of esophageal intubation.

2. Qualitative end-tidal CO_2 detection

Devices are now available that use a light indicator, such as a light-emitting diode (LED), to indicate an adequate concentration of CO_2 in exhaled air. These devices are very much analogous to the color-change indicators described earlier. The advantage of the LED system, which is often supplemented by an audible signal, is that they are more amenable to areas with poor lighting, such as in the prehospital setting. The small piece of the apparatus that actually inserts into the airway circuit is inexpensive and disposable. An audible alarm may sound when inadequate CO_2 is detected for a period of several seconds. The disadvantages of these devices are a greater capital outlay, and the potential for the devices to malfunction, lose power, or be stolen or misplaced. Nevertheless, they are reliable and accurate with the same precautions as those described earlier for the colorimetric devices.

3. Quantitative end-tidal CO_2 detection

The use of formal capnography allows the detection of CO_2 in the exhaled air to be recorded in a cyclical pattern on an ongoing basis. This provides information about ventilation, successful tube placement, and even underlying conditions and problems. Capnography is discussed in Chapter 30.

C. Aspiration techniques

Aspiration techniques involve the aspiration of a large volume of air rapidly through the ETT to determine whether the tube is in the trachea or the esophagus. The trachea is a rigid-walled structure and will permit the free flow of large volumes of air. The esophagus is a soft-sided structure, and attempts to aspirate large volumes of air quickly through an ETT will result in collapse of the esophageal walls against both the distal ETT orifice and the Murphy's eye. Aspiration devices are not as reliable as end-tidal CO_2 detection and should be considered as second-line devices for confirmation of tube placement. Two types of devices capitalize on the aspiration principle, bulb aspiration devices and syringe aspiration devices.

1. Bulb aspiration devices

Bulb aspiration devices consist of a round, compressible plastic globe, much like the compressible portion of a turkey baster, that is attached to a standard ETT adapter. The globe is held in the hand and compressed until flat, usually with the thumb. The deflated bulb is then placed firmly on the end of the ETT and the thumb is rapidly released, allowing the globe to reexpand, drawing a large quantity of air quickly through the ETT to do so. In the event of endotracheal placement of the tube, the bulb will immediately reexpand. Esophageal placement of the ETT will generally prevent reexpansion of the globe, although in some cases reexpansion will occur in a delayed fashion. It is recommended that reexpansion in under 2 seconds be taken as definitive evidence of tracheal placement and that failure of reexpansion within 30 seconds be taken as evidence of esophageal placement. Times between 2 and 30 seconds would be considered indeterminate. However, in virtually all cases of tracheal placement, immediate reinflation will occur. Any case in which immediate reinflation is not observed should be considered to be esophageal intubation until proven otherwise.

2. Syringe aspiration devices

Syringe aspiration devices use the same principle as bulb aspiration devices. A syringe aspiration device consists of a large syringe, usually 30 ml or more, affixed to a standard ETT adapter. Some devices also have ring-type adapters on the syringe plunger to facilitate easy aspiration. The device is placed on the ETT and the operator attempts extremely rapid aspiration of a large quantity of air by pulling back on the syringe plunger. Again, rapid easy flow of air indicates tracheal intubation, and resistance indicates esophageal intubation. As with the bulb aspiration device, any finding other than free-and-easy aspiration of air should be taken as evidence of esophageal intubation until proven otherwise.

II. Recommendations

Independent means of tube confirmation by end-tidal CO_2 detection are readily available, inexpensive, and highly reliable. It is recommended that such a device be used in every endotracheal intubation performed in the emergency department and that such devices be employed as a means of early assessment of ETT placement for those patients who arrive at the emergency department already intubated. End-tidal CO_2 detection can also be used with the Combitube. The aspiration detection devices have shown more variability in studies and cannot be considered as reliable as end-tidal CO_2 detection at present. Nevertheless, the aspiration devices may offer advantages over end-tidal CO_2 in certain circumstances, such as limited lighting in a prehospital setting. In all cases, end-tidal CO_2 should be evaluated, and if it is not clearly indicative of tracheal intubation, immediate action is indicated. If the patient is in prolonged cardiac arrest, insufficient CO_2 may be exchanged in the lungs, and direct laryngoscopy or an aspiration technique may be attempted. In all other cases, the ETT should be considered in the esophagus and the patient should be immediately reintubated.

ADDITIONAL READING

Murphy MF. Monitoring the emergency patient. In: Rosen P, Barkin R, Danzl DF, et al., eds. *Emergency medicine: concepts and clinical practice,* 4th ed. St Louis: Mosby, 1998.

Walls RM. Airway management. In: Rosen P, Barkin R, Danzl DF, et al., eds. *Emergency medicine: concepts and clinical practice,* 4th ed. St Louis: Mosby, 1998.

5

The Difficult and Failed Airway

Michael F. Murphy* and Ron M. Walls[†]

*Departments of Emergency Medicine and Anaesthesiology, Queen Elizabeth II
Health Sciences Centre, Dalhousie University, Halifax, Nova Scotia;
†Chairman, Department of Emergency Medicine, Brigham and Women's Hospital,
Associate Professor of Medicine, Division of Emergency Medicine,
Harvard Medical School, Boston, Massachusetts

The ability to manage an airway appropriately is fundamental to resuscitation. Failure to do so, particularly where that failure might have been predicted or avoided by the selection of a more appropriate technique, is disastrous. In the emergency department (ED), time frames are compressed, events are unpredictable, and conditions usually less than ideal. This emphasizes the need for emergency physicians to possess consummate airway evaluation and intervention skills.

An essential step in the evaluation of a patient for rapid sequence intubation (RSI) is the determination as to whether the patient has attributes that will make oral intubation, bag-and-mask ventilation, or airway rescue maneuvers difficult to achieve. Many airways are difficult to manage in the emergency setting, "difficulty" having three dimensions:

- Difficult to oxygenate and ventilate
- Difficult to intubate
- Difficult to perform a cricothyroidotomy

Sakles's depiction of the relationship among these dimensions as a triangle is shown in the Box 5.1. RSI represents the cognitive choice should the dimensions of difficulty be eliminated in the evaluation of the patient.

This chapter deals with the preemptive recognition of airway management difficulty. It is often possible to identify those patients where difficulty performing oral laryngoscopy and intubation will be encountered. Direct laryngoscopy is a key step in the identification process. The individual managing the airway must be able to assess and anticipate the degree of difficulty and then select a method of airway management most likely to succeed, rather than embarking on a path destined to fail.

It has been estimated that between 1% and 3% of patients present with difficult airways leading to difficult endotracheal intubation under direct vision using a laryngoscope. The anesthesia literature tells us that intubation will fail between 0.1% and 0.4% of the time in patients assessed as likely to be successfully intubated. The chance that a patient will be unpredictably impossible to intubate or ventilate with a bag and mask approaches 1 in 10,000. These statistics are derived from elective anesthesia practice. Airway management failure in the ED is probably more common. In the 1,288 patients reported during the pilot phase of the National Emergency Airway Registry (NEAR), the incidence of "rescue" cricothyrotomy was 1%.

The single most important factor in dictating success or failure in airway management is the airway manager, who must be familiar with an array of airway management equipment and

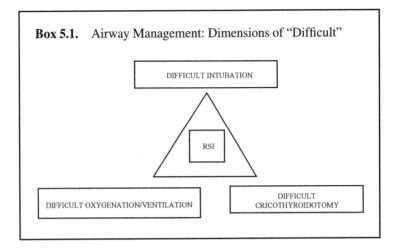

Box 5.1. Airway Management: Dimensions of "Difficult"

DIFFICULT INTUBATION

RSI

DIFFICULT OXYGENATION/VENTILATION

DIFFICULT CRICOTHYROIDOTOMY

must be able to select and use them appropriately. Armed with this knowledge and skill, the airway manager can plan for difficulty and respond appropriately to failure, should it occur. A detailed knowledge of the medications used to facilitate intubation, especially the contraindications and complications attendant with their use, is essential. Not all airway management failures are avoidable. The goal is to minimize the potential for disastrous outcomes.

Anticipating the difficult intubation and selecting the appropriate technique to secure the airway reduces the incidence of failed intubation. Successful application of these principles is predicated on three pillars:

- Recognizing and predicting the difficult intubation
- Choosing the most appropriate technique and equipment for the particular situation
- Possessing a comprehensive set of pharmacologic and technical skills and the necessary drugs and devices to succeed.

I. The difficult airway
A. Predicting the difficult airway
It is unusual for an emergency intubation to allow the luxury of a detailed patient interview prior to the procedure. The emergency physician may be able to ascertain a prior history of airway management difficulty rapidly from individuals accompanying the patient or from other sources, such as a MedicAlert bracelet.
1. Anatomic features
- One of the first clues to difficult intubation or ventilation may come from simple visual inspection of the patient. Morbid obesity predicts difficult intubation, difficult ventilation, and rapid oxygen desaturation. Abnormal facial shape, facial or neck trauma, large teeth, protruding tongue, or presence of facial hair may portend difficult intubation, ventilation, or both.
- All false teeth, especially full upper or lower dentures, should be removed prior to intubation. Large upper incisors may obstruct visualization of the larynx. Protruding upper incisors reduce visualization and access because they elongate the anteroposterior axis of the mouth, as does a large mandible. Jagged teeth may lacerate the balloons on ETTs or Combitubes.
- Patients with narrow facial features and high-arched palates may have a difficult airway. Access to the airway is limited because of the reduced space from side to side in the mouth. In addition, the longer anteroposterior dimension limits the ability to visualize the larynx.

2. Physical examination of the airway

- An adult with normal Temperomandibular Joint (TMJ) function ought to be able to open the mouth to accommodate three fingers (3 to 4 cm) incisor to incisor, top to bottom.
- The mandible ought to be sufficiently large to accommodate a normal-sized tongue. In the adult, one should expect three finger-breadths space between the tip of the chin (mentum) and the hyoid bone. A patient with a small mandible will have a tongue that obstructs access to the larynx during intubation (i.e., the larynx is tucked up under the base of the tongue). Also, a dimension greatly exceeding three fingers elongates the oral axis (one of the three to be aligned during orotracheal intubation), making it more difficult to bring it into alignment with the larynx.
- The length of the neck and the position of the larynx in the neck are also important. The larynx descends in the neck from the C3,4 level in infancy to the C5,6 level by 8 or 9 years of age. A larynx that is higher (e.g., in morbid obesity) may be more difficult to visualize at the time of orotracheal intubation than one that is lower, as it is tucked up under the base of the tongue.
- Typically, one ought to be able to get two fingers between the top of the thyroid cartilage and the floor of the mouth in a normal adult (Box 5.2)

3. The Mallampati score and grade of laryngeal view

Airway management difficulty is best predicted by performing the following maneuver: With the patient seated, have him or her extend the neck, open the mouth as far as possible, and protrude the tongue as far as possible. Observe the degree to which the base of the tongue, faucial pillars, uvula, and posterior pharynx are visible. A four-point scale is used to describe the degree to which visualization is possible (Mallampati, Fig. 5.1). A grade 1 view provides a view of the entire posterior oropharynx, to the bases of the tonsillar pillars. A grade 4 view permits no visualization of the posterior oropharynx with the tongue totally obstructing visualization of the uvula. Oropharyngeal visualization correlates with laryngeal visualization. Grade 1 and 2 Mallampati views are associated with superior laryngeal exposure (Fig. 5.1) by conventional laryngoscopy (laryngeal grades 1 and 2) at the time of intubation and with low intubation failure rates. Grade 3 and 4 views, on the other hand, are associated with increasingly poor laryngeal visualization (laryngeal grades 3 and 4) and with higher intubation failure rates. This formal version of the maneuver is seldom possible or practical in the ED, though examination of the supine patient with a tongue blade may prove useful.

4. Airway obstruction

- Even in the absence of any other predictors of difficult intubation, upper-airway obstruction may make intubation and ventilation difficult or impossible. For ex-

---

Box 5.2. The 3-3-2 rule

For the purpose of easy recall, we call this three-finger mouth-opening, three-finger mentum-to-hyoid, and two-finger floor-of-mouth-to-thyroid cartilage the "3-3-2 rule" and rapidly use it to assess the external dimensions of the airway and predict difficulty.

Mallampati Signs as Indicators
of Difficult Intubation

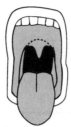

Class I: soft palate, uvula,
fauces, pillars visible

No difficulty

Class II: soft palate,
uvula, fauces visible

No difficulty

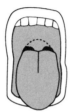

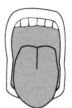

Class III: soft palate, base
of uvula visible

Moderate difficulty

Class IV: hard palate
only visible

Severe difficulty

FIG. 5.1. The Mallampati Score for prediction of difficulty in intubation. (KW Publications, with permission.)

ample, the otherwise anatomically normal 20-year-old man with epiglottitis will be difficult to intubate for that reason alone. Similarly, the trauma patient with a midneck hematoma may be difficult or impossible to intubate or ventilate because of intrusion by the hematoma.

- The obstructed or distorted airway is discussed in detail elsewhere in this manual.

5. **Cervical spine mobility**
   - C-spine immobilization adds a dimension of difficulty to the airway management scenario, as it reduces one's ability to align the necessary axes in facilitating orotracheal intubation. As an aside, it also affects the performance of Sellick's maneuver, as the application of cricoid pressure has the potential of causing motion of the unstable segments. However, Sellick's maneuver is still recommended in patients with possible cervical spine injury.
   - Patients with decreased cervical spine mobility caused by disease, such as rheumatoid arthritis, may be difficult or impossible to intubate because of inability to position the head and neck in a way that aligns the axes of intubation.

B. **The LEMON Law**

Although numerous physical features, measurements and scores have been advocated as useful in identifying airway management difficulty, none have proved to be failsafe in predicting intubation failure, and none have undergone rigorous scientific evaluation in an ED setting. Time pressures and the reality of the ED setting require any airway evaluation to be simple and easily remembered. Through many iterations the developers of the National Emergency Airway Management Course have developed the "LEMON Law" for identification of the difficult airway (Box 5.3). Although yet to be scientifically validated, it is a common sense approach well suited to the ED setting and covers all the airway evaluations outlined above.

Look externally. The patient should be examined for characteristics that identify either difficult intubation or difficult ventilation. For example, the presence of a beard or moustache may hinder adequate mask seal and make bag ventilation difficult. An abnormal facial shape, extreme cachexia, an edentulous mouth with sunken cheeks, or disruption of the lower face by trauma may make adequate mask seal and bag ventilation very difficult. Large central incisors or "buck" teeth and a high-arching palate, receding mandible, or short bull neck may make oral intubation difficult. Obesity may make both intubation and ventilation more difficult. Thus the first step in the evaluation of the difficult airway is to look for external characteristics that would predict difficult intubation or difficult ventilation.

Evaluate the 3-3-2 rule. The geometry of oral intubation requires alignment of the oral axis, the pharyngeal axis, and the laryngeal axis to permit access to the trachea. The 3-3-2 rule evaluates these relationships. The first step in the 3-3-2 rule is to place three fingers between the patient's teeth; in other words, the patient's mouth should open adequately to permit three fingers to be placed between the upper and lower teeth. The second 3 of the 3-3-2 rule involves measurement of the space from the mentum to the hyoid bone. Again, three fingers placed side by side should fit in this space. This identifies adequate mandibular dimension to permit access to the airway. The 2 in the 3-3-2 rule requires that two fingers be placed between the thyroid notch and the floor of the mouth (i.e. the hyoid bone). This indicates that the larynx is sufficiently low within the neck to permit access by the oral route. Thus the 3-3-2 rule, which is easily remembered, is three fingers into the mouth, three fingers under the chin, and two fingers at the top of the neck (patients own fingers).

Mallampati. The Mallampati classification is an indication of the amount of space available within the mouth to accomodate both the laryngoscope and an endotracheal tube. The Mallampati classification is performed by having the patient open the mouth as wide as possible and stick the tongue out. This is ideally done in the sitting position with the head protruding forward, mimicking the "sniffing" position for intubation. In the ED, this is rarely possible. The Mallampati evaluation is often done with the patient supine, and may, in fact, be done with a tongue blade as an estimation in the unresponsive patient. The four Mallampati grades are shown in Fig. 5.1 and range from class I, identifying excellent oral access, through class IV, which identifies very difficult oral access and thus difficult intubation.

Obstruction? Obstruction of the upper airway will lead to difficulty both with intubation and with ventilation. If the patient has a known laryngeal tumor, known or sus-

---

Box 5.3. The LEMON law

For difficult airway assessment
L   *L*ook externally
E   *E*valuate the 3-3-2 rule
M   *M*allampati
O   *O*bstruction?
N   *N*eck mobility

pected epiglottitis, known or suspected peritonsillar abscess, known or suspected prevertebral abscess, or any other condition of the upper airway that might result in obstruction, then both laryngoscopy and bag ventilation may be rendered difficult. The presence of a foreign body, direct airway trauma, extrinsic airway hematoma with compression, or possible disruption of the integrity of the airway should be considered evidence of obstruction that may render intubation and ventilation difficult or impossible.

Neck mobility. One of the most important attributes necessary for successful intubation or ventilation is the ability for the patient's head and neck to be positioned adequately to permit laryngeal access via the oral cavity. Neck mobility is frequently reduced, especially in elderly patients and those with systemic arthritides. A good test for neck mobility in the cooperative patient is to ask the patient in the sitting position to look at the floor. The patient should be instructed to put the chin right down on the chest and look downward. The patient should then be asked to bring the head and neck all the way up to look upward at the ceiling behind the head. As he or she does this, the patient will pass the head and neck through an arc representing the sniffing position for intubation. In the uncooperative patient, a quick check of neck mobility will prevent later grief. Obviously, the immobilized trauma patient automatically presents a difficult airway because of neck immobilization, but in such cases, oral intubation is almost always successful in the absence of other difficult airway attributes.

Thus a systematic approach to the difficult airway consists of evaluation of the LEMON attributes and assessment of their impact on airway management and ventilation.

II. Clinical approach to the difficult airway

The difficult airway algorithm is discussed in detail in Chapter 3. Some points deserve emphasis in this chapter (Fig. 5.2).

A. Step D-1: Difficult airway predicted

If airway management is predicted to be difficult, the old adage that "nothing should be taken from the patient that the airway manager cannot replace" provides a good reference point. This applies particularly to the administration of paralytic drugs. Also, some patient circumstances mandate prompt intubation even in the presence of a difficult airway. Nowhere in emergency medicine are skills, experience, and judgment more important.

B. Step D-4: Bag-and-mask ventilation predicted to be successful?

In other words, if intubation fails, will bag-and-mask ventilation be possible? One must have a high degree of certainty to answer this question in the affirmative, particularly if one is contemplating the use of paralytic agents. Various anatomic and physiologic factors may predict the likelihood of failure, as described above.

C. Step D-4-1: Intubation predicted to be successful?

The decision to proceed with RSI in the patient with a predicted difficult airway must be attended by a high degree of certainty that it will be successful. The airway manager must be confident and possess a broad array of equipment and skills to rescue the airway in the event that conventional direct-vision orotracheal intubation fails.

D. Step D-5: Topical anesthesia, sedation, and "awake" laryngoscopy

These techniques comprise those that use sedative agents, topical anesthetic agents, or usually both, to blunt airway reflexes and patient responses so that a "trial" laryngoscopy can be performed, without abolishing the patient's native respiratory drive or airway patency. The condition of the patient and the clinical situation will dictate the comprehensiveness of this maneuver. (How much does one need to see?) It may be

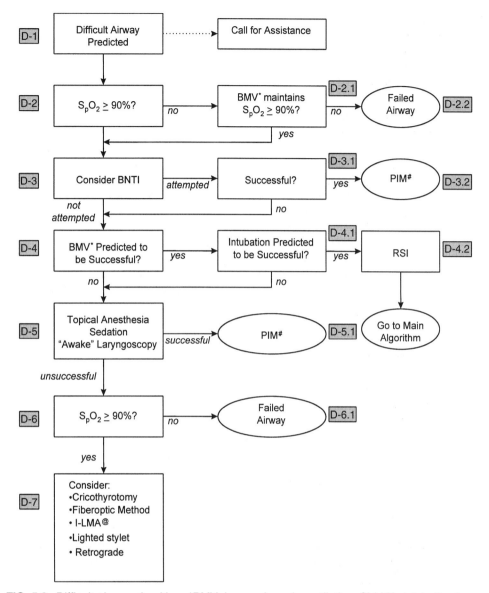

FIG. 5.2. Difficult airway algorithm. *BMV, bag-and-mask ventilation; @I-LMA, intubating laryngeal mask airway; #PIM, postintubation (FASTRACH) management.

that the airway manager simply needs to verify that the epiglottis is in the midline to make the decision to back off and move to RSI. At other times, it may progress to an awake intubation. The rule of thumb is that if the condition that is causing the difficult intubation is the same one that mandates intubation (i.e., an acute, dynamic process), then if the vocal cords are visualized during awake laryngoscopy, intubation should be achieved right then. However, if a patient with a chronic (nonchanging) difficult airway condition requires intubation because of a separate, acute process, visualization of the glottis during awake laryngoscopy may be used to support a decision to proceed with controlled RSI.

III. The failed airway
  A. Definition
    There are many definitions of the failed airway. Most use the number of unsuccessful attempts (e.g., two or three) to define failure. However, in clinical practice the definition is multifactorial and needs to integrate the following:
      1. Number of failed attempts (e.g., three);
      2. Ability to ventilate the patient with a bag and mask;
      3. Ability to maintain reasonable oxygen saturations;
      4. Ability to visualize the larynx.
    For example, attempts to secure the anatomically disrupted airway (e.g., gun shot wound (GSW) face) in the face of an inability to maintain a patent airway or reasonable saturations would likely be defined as a failure after a single attempt and motivate the emergency physician to move immediately to a surgical airway.
      Clinically, the failed airway may be one of two types:
      1. Cannot intubate but can oxygenate with a bag-and-mask device.
      2. Cannot intubate and cannot oxygenate.
    The National Emergency Airway Management Course defines *failure* simply:
      1. Failure to intubate on three attempts by a skilled and experienced operator. This is called the "can't intubate, can oxygenate" failure.
      2. Any failure to intubate, no matter the number of attempts, in the face of oxygen saturations that cannot be maintained at 90% or higher using a bag and mask. This is called the "can't intubate, can't oxygenate" scenario.

  B. Management
    The failed-airway algorithm is presented in Chapter 3. Most often, in the "can't intubate but can oxygenate" situation, the conventional direct-vision orotracheal intubation technique has failed, though one is at least able to maintain reasonable ventilation and oxygenation while planning additional strategies. In this type of case, the airway manager has the time to consider alternative techniques, such as the following:
    • A light-guided technique
    • Retrograde intubation
    • The intubating laryngeal mask (ILM)
    • Fiberoptic techniques
    Little information is currently available to support a recommendation of one technique over the other in the management of the failed airway. An approach should be dictated by the operator's expertise and experience, available equipment, and patient attributes.
      The continuous application of cricoid pressure may serve to minimize the risk of aspiration and gastric distension in this instance.
      The second situation, in which one can neither intubate nor oxygenate, is considerably more desperate and is addressed in one of two ways:
      1. Cricothyrotomy. If a surgical airway is not immediately achievable, the use of an airway adjunct such as a Combitube or a laryngeal mask should be attempted provided the airway obstruction is not at or below the level of the larynx. The ILM may permit successful tracheal intubation.
      2. The use of a percutaneous transtracheal jet ventilator (PTTV) as a temporizing measure if laryngeal patency is assured.

IV. Conclusions
  Prepare in advance for failure, particularly in the ED, where
  • Time frames are compressed and detailed airway evaluation is impossible.
  • Complex airway problems occur with predictable frequency.

Remember that

- The first response to a failure of bag-and-mask ventilation is better bag-and-mask ventilation. Insert nasal airways in both nostrils and an oral airway in the mouth. Optimize airway position by thrusting the mandible forward and holding it there. Use a two-handed mask hold; try picking the head up off the pillow to open the airway if the C-spine is alright.
- Use judicious sedation and topical airway anesthesia to have a quick look if a difficult laryngoscopy is predicted.
- Generate as much positive pressure as possible without inflating the stomach.
- Consider using sedative and paralytic agents to increase the chances of success in selected circumstances.

ADDITIONAL READING

Benumof JL, ed. *Airway management and clinical practice.* St Louis: Mosby, 1996

Benumof JL. Management of the difficult adult airway. *Anesthesiology* 1991;75:1087.

Bogdonoff DL, Bogdonoff DL, Stone DJ. Emergency management of the airway outside the operating room. *Can J Anaesth* 1992;39:1069

Crosby ET. The adult cervical spine: implications for airway management. *Can J Anaesth* 1990;37:77.

Dailey RH, ed. *The airway: emergency management.* St Louis: Mosby, 1992.

Finucane BT, Santora AH. Principles of airway management. In: Lowenthal DT, ed. Essentials of Medical Education Series. Ed. Philadelphia: FA Davis, 1988.

Lewis M, Kermati S, Benumoff JL, et al. What is the best way to determine oropharyngeal classification and mandibular space length to predict difficult laryngoscopy. *Anesthesiology* 1994;81:69.

Lyons G. Failed intubation: six years experience in a maternity unit. *Anaesthesia* 1985;40:759.

Mallampati SR, Gatt SP, Gugino LD, et al. A clinical sign to predict difficult intubation: a prospective study. *Can Anesth Soc J* 1985;32:429.

McIntyre JWR. The difficult tracheal intubation *Can J Anaesth* 1987;34:204.

Meschino A, Devitt JH, Koch JP, et al. The safety of awake tracheal intubation in cervical spine injury *Can J Anaesth* 1992;39:114.

Miller RD, ed. *Anesthesia,* 2nd ed. New York: Churchill Livingstone, 1986.

Norton ML, Brown ACD. *Atlas of the Difficult Airway.* St Louis: Mosby Year Book, 1991.

Oates JDL, Macleod AD, Oates PD, et al. Comparison of two methods for predicting difficult intubation. *Br J Anaesth* 1991;66:305.

Practice Guidelines for Management of the Difficult Airway. ASA task force report. *Anesthesiology* 1993;78:597.

Rose EK, Cohen MM. The airway: problems and predictions in 18,500 patients. *Can J Anaesth* 1994;41:372.

Samsoon GLT, et al. Difficult tracheal intubation: a retrospective review. *Anaesthesia* 1987;42:487.

Suderman VS, Crosby ET, Lai A. Elective oral tracheal intubation in cervical spine injured adults. *Can J Anaesth* 1991;38:785.

SECTION 2

Airway Management Techniques

6

Basic Airway Management

Robert E. Schneider

Carolinas Medical Center, Department of Emergency Medicine,
Charlotte, North Carolina

Although all airway skills are important, perhaps the most important skill is the ability to use a bag and mask along with upper-airway adjuncts to ventilate a patient. This is known as basic airway management. Substantial skill is required to maintain an adequate mask seal, position the head, and assure a patent airway with one hand while ventilating with the other. Once mastered, however, this technique reduces both the urgency to intubate and the anxiety that universally accompanies a failed intubation attempt. This is especially true if muscle relaxants have been used to facilitate intubation. Bag-and-mask ventilation is a reasonable airway adjunct for short periods of time, provided one takes steps to minimize the risk of aspiration of gastric contents. In fact, competence with bag-and-mask ventilation is a prerequisite to using paralytic agents to intubate the trachea.

I. Technique

1. Select and insert the appropriate upper-airway adjuncts: a nasopharyngeal airway to ensure patency of the posterior nasopharynx if active upper-airway reflexes are intact; an oropharyngeal airway to control the tongue if upper-airway reflexes are absent. Both may be required in selected circumstances (see items 8 and 9 in this list) and are mandatory to achieve optimum bag-and-mask ventilation.

2. If possible, position the head and neck in the "sniffing the morning air" position. A pillow or towel under the occiput and extension of the head on the neck will facilitate parallel alignment of the oral, pharyngeal, and laryngeal axes. The need to maintain a neutral C-spine position in the patient with suspected C-spine injury adds an element of difficulty to opening and maintaining the airway.

3. The airway manager must be able to evaluate the effectiveness of bag-and-mask ventilation. This is accomplished by feeling the resistance in the bag, watching the chest rise and fall, ensuring that air does not enter the stomach, and monitoring oxygen saturation. A bag should be selected that is able to deliver high pressure, especially in children. A soft bag allows the operator to appreciate compliance and resistance while squeezing the bag. The addition of a variable, positive-pressure relief valve in the circuit allows one to adjust the amount of positive pressure in the system. Conventional self-inflating bags (e.g., Laerdal) may incorporate defeatable positive-pressure relief valves, but the design of the bag does not allow the care provider to develop the same "feel" for compliance and resistance during ventilation.

4. Place the mask initially on the nasal bridge and then lever it down onto the malar eminences and alveolar ridge, covering the nose and mouth. The mask may be maneuvered superiorly or inferiorly to achieve the best fit.

5. The thumb and index finger are used to apply pressure to the mask and obtain a seal on the face. It may be necessary to rock the mask up or down, or from side to side, or to gather the cheek inside the mask to achieve an adequate seal. It is easier to get an adequate mask seal if the mask is too large than it is if it is too small. In masks with inflatable collars, ensure that the collar is inflated with the correct amount of air, as collars that are over- or underinflated may be more difficult to seal.

6. The long, ring, and little fingers are maximally abducted to capture as much of the mandible as possible. Usually, the little finger is placed under the angle of the mandible, allowing the operator to thrust the mandible forward. The long finger is placed under the mandibular symphysis and in conjunction with the ring and little fingers is used to lift the chin and thrust the jaw forward, opening the airway. From time to time it may be necessary to remove the bag and mask and use both hands to open the mouth slightly and thrust the jaw forward. Maintaining this jaw position will keep the airway open while bag-and-mask ventilation is resumed.

7. In difficult situations, it may be necessary for one person to use both hands to open the airway and ensure a good mask seal. This can be done by placing the thenar eminences along the superior ridge of the mask and strategically placing the remaining abducted four fingers from both hands along the body and angles of the mandible to ensure jaw thrust and airway patency. A modification of this technique is to place the index fingers and thumbs of both hands in apposition to one another along the inferior and superior ridges of the mask and use the remaining abducted three fingers for jaw thrust. The former method is recommended because it is more comfortable, and the thenar eminences are stronger and will fatigue much later than the index fingers. In desperate situations, a single care provider can achieve ventilation by squeezing the bag between his or her elbow and chest/lateral abdomen or between his or her knees while using both hands to optimize the mask seal until help can be recruited.

8. When initial or standard bag-and-mask ventilation fails to establish or maintain adequate oxygen saturation, one should immediately review the following options:
   - Is the patient in the optimum sniffing position? If not, how can the position be improved?
   - Are all upper-airway adjuncts properly utilized? Can a nasal or oral airway or both be deployed?
   - Is the mask seal optimal? If not, how can this be improved (e.g., applying KY jelly to a beard; placing unfolded gauze 4×4s fluffed and compressed inside the mouth along the buccal pouches (cheeks) to create a more anatomically normal mask seal; reinserting the patient's false teeth).
   - Can another person be recruited to help optimize bag-and-mask technique?

9. In situations where attempts at bag-and-mask ventilation are unsuccessful, better bag-and-mask techniques must be employed. Bag-and-mask ventilation should not be abandoned until optimum bag-and-mask techniques have been utilized and have proven ineffective. This requires placing the patient in the optimum sniffing position, placing an oral airway and two nasopharyngeal airways, and using two care providers, one to facilitate optimum mask seal with aggressive action to ensure that the mandible is displaced in a forward direction and another to squeeze the bag.

10. In the patient with spontaneous ventilatory efforts, open the airway and evaluate the adequacy of gas exchange. If partial or complete obstruction persists, provide continuous positive airway pressure, as this may simultaneously open the airway and allow adequate, spontaneous, patient-generated ventilation. In the face of persistent airway

obstruction or ventilatory inadequacy, it may be necessary to coordinate synchronous bag-and-mask ventilation with the patient's respiratory effort to maintain or augment gas exchange. This sounds easy in theory but can be difficult to master because failure to synchronize efforts may exacerbate inadequate gas exchange, lead to gastric distension, and increase the risk of regurgitation and aspiration.

11. In most clinical settings pulse oximetry reflects adequate oxygenation but provides no information regarding the adequacy of ventilation and carbon dioxide elimination. Clinical judgment is paramount in assessing the adequacy of ventilation.

II. Laryngoscopy and intubation

Direct laryngoscopy is the centerpiece of orotracheal intubation. In most situations, the laryngoscopy technique itself, coupled with the intubator's skill, makes the difference between a successful intubation or progression to a failed airway. Laryngoscopy is a learned skill, and when it is performed properly, it provides optimal exposure of the glottic opening, facilitating endotracheal intubation. Laryngoscopy is a multifaceted procedure that requires both dexterity and creativity to align the unparalleled oral, pharyngeal, and laryngeal axes of the airway so that the laryngoscopist will be provided the best possible view. Unfortunately, the actual technique of laryngoscopy seems to generate little attention during medical education. Emergency medicine residents are systematically trained in intubation, both in the operating room and in the emergency department, but the essential elements of laryngoscopy are often covered superficially, with more time devoted to drugs and alternative methods of intubation. Many practicing clinicians have had little formal training in laryngoscopy and do not have a clear, intuitive understanding of the geometry involved and the subsequent anatomic manipulation that can predictably improve glottic visualization. Because there are many different techniques of laryngoscopy, the laryngoscopist must choose one method that works best and use or practice it often. The paraglossal technique of laryngoscopy presented in this chapter is safe, quick, reproducible, and can be used universally with either a curved or straight blade in both children and adults. Even a relatively inexperienced practitioner can achieve competence with this technique if the principles and sequential steps are fully understood and regularly practiced.

A. Anatomy of intubation

To appreciate the intricacies of laryngoscopy, one must first understand the anatomy of the larynx, how to handle the laryngoscope, how to select the best blade for the patient at hand, and how to maneuver the patient and his or her laryngeal anatomy into the optimum position to provide the best view of the vocal cords.

In the larynx, the vocal cords, which define the glottic opening, lie inferior and posterior to the flexible epiglottis, which emanates from the hyoid bone and base of the tongue. During laryngoscopy, these constant relationships serve as important anatomic landmarks. When in trouble, one *must* find the epiglottis, because usually it leads to the airway. There will be occasions during routine or difficult laryngoscopy when the esophagus is exposed and mistaken for the vocal cords. Unless one has a landmark or consistent reference point to confirm the airway anatomically, esophageal intubation may ensue or intubation may be unsuccessful. Whenever one is uncertain whether the visualized opening is the glottis or the esophagus, the laryngoscope should be withdrawn until the tip of the superiorly compressed epiglottis falls into view. Once identified, the tip of the epiglottis can usually be elevated with either the straight or curved blade exposing the cords and the arytenoid cartilages, allowing confident placement of the endotracheal tube (ETT) into the airway.

The single greatest obstacle to successful laryngoscopy is the tongue. To the laryngoscopist, the tongue is the enemy. Anatomically, the base of the tongue may block access to the glottic opening. When the tongue is large in relation to the oral cavity (Mallampati class 3 or 4), it can inhibit adequate exposure of the glottic aperture. For this reason, preintubation assessment of the patient's airway is essential. The method emphasized in this

manual uses the mnemonic LEMON (Chapter 5). The *M* (Mallampati) in *LEMON* is a re-
minder to examine the oral cavity to assess the relative size of the tongue in relationship to
the oropharynx and to allow assessment regarding tongue mobility and potential glottic exposure during laryngoscopy. The laryngoscope blade is the tool that controls and maneuvers the tongue. In general, the larger the tongue, the wider the blade (i.e., #3 or #4) that
should be selected. One of the basic tenets in successful laryngoscopy is to select a blade,
curved or straight, that will be wide and long enough to capture the tongue and sweep it
leftward, out of the visual field, thus allowing direct visual access to the airway (Fig. 6.1).

B. Technique of laryngoscopy

In the emergent situation, it is important to have a technique of laryngoscopy that is
simple, consistent, universal (i.e., it can be used for curved or straight blade intubations
in pediatric or adult patients), and applicable to virtually every clinical situation. Laryngoscopy is not about strength or muscle power, but about finesse and the ability to "feel"
the tip of the advancing laryngoscope. The paraglossal technique is one in which the
entire length of the laryngoscope blade is inserted blindly but gently into the esophagus, then slowly withdrawn, under vision, most often exposing the cords first, then the
epiglottis, which can be picked up with the tip of either blade, providing maximum laryngeal exposure for successful intubation. The traditional technique of inserting a
curved blade into the vallecula may be more difficult, tends to be more traumatic, and
may be less effective at consistently locating important landmarks.

The first stage of laryngoscopy is nonvisual (i.e., the entire laryngoscope blade is passed
not under direct vision but by feel and appreciation of the oral, pharyngeal, and esophageal
anatomy). The second stage, or active stage of laryngoscopy, is totally visual. It may require
transient muscle power just before intubation to achieve the last bit of glottic exposure.

The laryngoscope should always be grasped in the left hand, unless an anatomic or neuromuscular abnormality in the laryngoscopist precludes this. The laryngoscope is held
with the fingers and thumb, not clenched in the palm of the hand. The handle of the laryngoscope should be grasped on one side with the fingertips of the index through fifth fingers, while the volar pad of the thumb is positioned on the opposite side (Fig. 6.2).

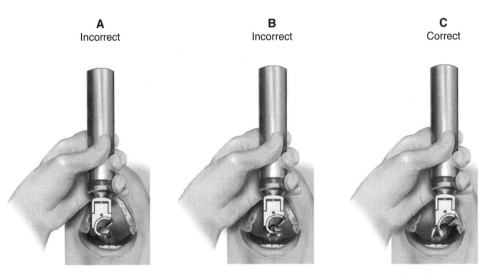

| **A** | **B** | **C** |
| Incorrect | Incorrect | Correct |

FIG. 6.1. Tongue control during laryngoscopy. **A** and **B** demonstrate poor visualization of the
cords due to incorrect positioning of the blade. Note how the tongue folds over the blade and
obscures the view. **C** demonstrates correct positioning of the blade to control and move the
tongue to the left, providing an optimal view for intubation.

Holding the laryngoscope handle in the palm of the hand and applying constant, firm muscle power throughout laryngoscopy, the "deathgrip," is not recommended, because it impairs technique and promotes muscle fatigue. At various times during laryngoscopy, transient, controlled muscle power may be required to negotiate the anatomic curvature of the posterior pharynx or gain additional glottic exposure to improve the view and allow successful passage of the ETT. Constant handgrip and forearm tension throughout laryngoscopy will quickly lead to muscle fatigue and impotence just when strength may be required to achieve the best view.

The laryngoscopist's right hand must remain free at all times and must not succumb to the habit of holding the ETT while initiating laryngoscopy. The right hand will be used for optimal positioning of the patient's head to achieve the sniffing position, for suctioning, for application of the BURP maneuver (see later), and for picking up or receiving the ETT when intubating the patient.

The first step in initiating laryngoscopy is to position the head and neck in the best possible anatomic position. In the trauma victim, where in-line stabilization of the cervical spine is recommended, or in patients with decreased cervical spine mobility, flexion of the lower cervical spine and extension of the head may be impossible or

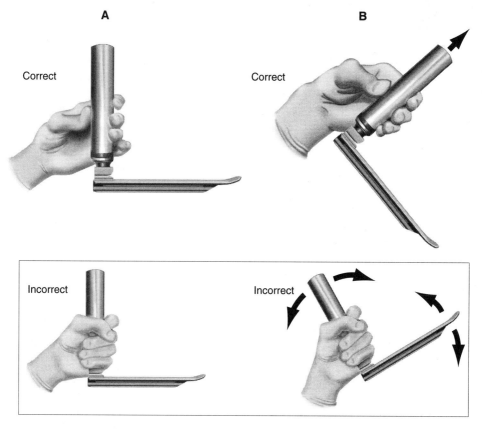

FIG. 6.2. Laryngoscopy. **A:** Recommended grip of the laryngoscope. **B:** Technique of achieving greater glottic exposure. Note how the end of the laryngoscope handle is directed at approximately 45 degrees and pull is applied longitudinally. **C:** Absence of the rocking motion will prevent dental injury and airway trauma.

inappropriate. An anatomically "neutral position" must be maintained in all patients with suspected cervical spine injury, thus making laryngoscopy more difficult (Fig. 6.3A). Patients with advanced cervical arthritis may have markedly reduced neck motion, which will also confound laryngoscopy. In all other patients, before placing the laryngoscope into the patient's mouth, the "sniffing" position is created by placing a pillow, folded towel, or sheet under the patient's head to facilitate forward flexion of the lower

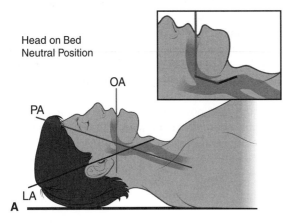

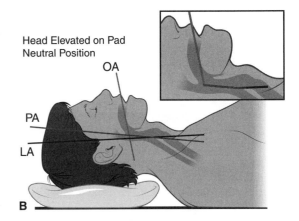

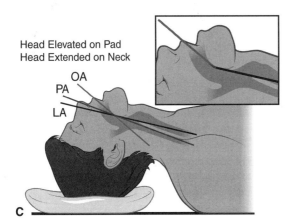

FIG. 6.3. A: Anatomic neutral position. The oral (OA), pharyngeal (PA), and laryngeal (LA) axes are at greater angles to one another. **B:** Head, still in neutral position, has been lifted by a pillow flexing the lower cervical spine and aligning the pharyngeal (PA) and laryngeal (LA) axes. **C:** The head has been extended on the cervical spine, aligning the oral axis (OA) with the pharyngeal (PA) and laryngeal (LA) axes, creating the optimum "sniffing" position for intubation. **D:** Relatively anteriorly placed larynx. **E:** BURP maneuver on the thyroid cartilage. **F:** BURP maneuver improves the laryngeal view for intubation.

cervical spine (Fig. 6.3B). Active extension of the head on the neck with the laryngo-scopist's right hand at the initiation of laryngoscopy should complete the ideal parallel alignment of the oral, pharyngeal, and laryngeal axes (Fig. 6.3C). These axes originate at almost 90-degree angles to one another in the neutral position (Fig. 6.3A). Creation of this parallel alignment of the axes produces the "sniffing" position and provides the optimum view of the cords, promoting successful intubation (Fig. 6.3).

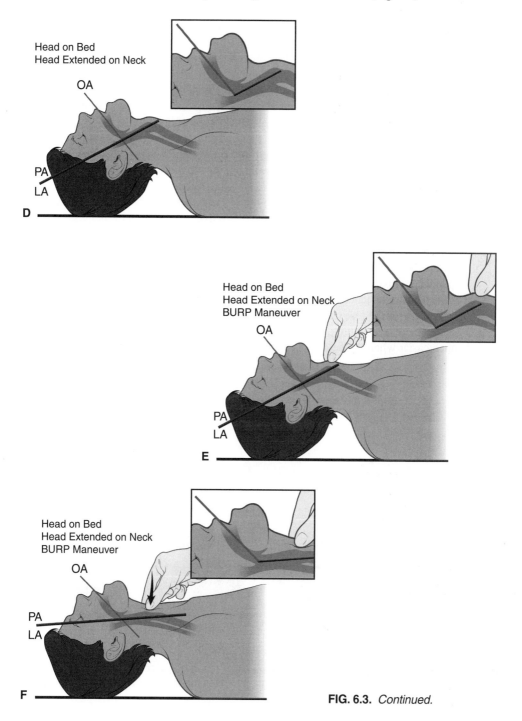

FIG. 6.3. *Continued.*

Once the optimal position for laryngoscopy has been achieved, the lower jaw is opened to gain access to the oropharynx. It is a matter of personal preference whether one wishes to utilize the scissor technique of opening the mouth or simply to grasp the mandible with the thumb, index, and long fingers of the right hand and open the mouth. The latter technique allows the laryngoscopist to retract the lower lip, providing full exposure of the mandibular teeth and the entire oropharynx. Assuming the patient is totally paralyzed with maximum mandibular mobility, the laryngoscope blade is placed into the patient's mouth. The flanged surface of the laryngoscope blade is carefully placed alongside the lingual surface (paraglossal) of the right mandibular molar teeth. This is an extremely important initial anatomic relationship in controlling the tongue (Fig. 6.4). The laryngoscopist must be certain there is no tongue between the flanged surface of the blade and the lingual surface of the mandibular molar teeth before initiating laryngoscopy. Failure to establish this starting position will compromise control of the tongue and visualization of the glottic aperture (Figs. 6.1 and 6.4).

Once the blade has been correctly positioned adjacent to the right mandibular molar teeth, its entire length is blindly passed into the patient's esophagus. This is accomplished by following the anatomic curvature of the tongue while moving the blade from the rightward lateral starting position to a slightly more midline position as the blade automatically traverses the base of the tongue and posterior pharynx, and then passes totally into the cervical esophagus (Fig 6.5). Active visualization of the posterior pharyngeal or laryngeal anatomy is neither required nor possible during this maneuver. The esophageal insertion is done completely by feel, with the gentle pressure exerted by the volar pads of the fingers and thumb allowing the laryngoscopist to "feel" the advancing tip of the laryngoscopic blade. The thumb should actually be placed on the proximal end of the blade at its junction with the handle to push the blade gently into the esophagus. Any perception of resistance during this maneuver requires immediate cessation of advancement, slight withdrawal with realignment, then reinsertion. This maneuver is much easier when the patient is in the "sniffing" position rather than the neutral posi-

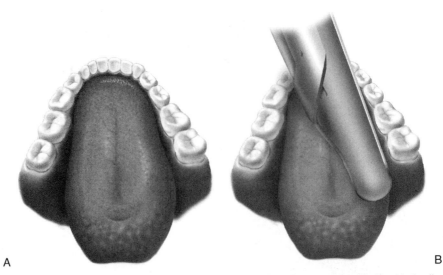

A   B

FIG. 6.4. A: Oral cavity. **B:** Initial anatomic relationship of the flange of the blade with the lingual surface of the molar teeth. Note there is no tongue between the flange of the blade and the teeth.

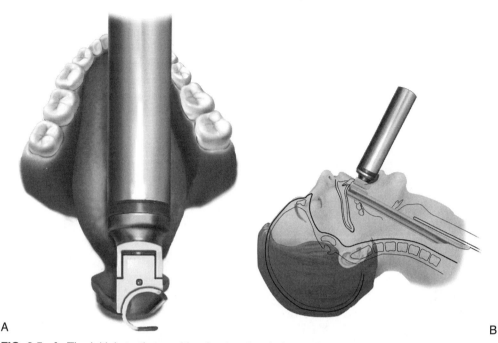

A   B

FIG. 6.5. A: The initial starting position for the visual phase of laryngoscopy. **B:** Note that the blade is in the esophagus and the blade/handle junction is at the patient's teeth. Note the position of the cords proximal to the tip of the blade.

tion. In the latter situation (most trauma patients), the laryngoscope blade must hug the anterior surface of the tongue as it is advanced atraumatically through the oropharynx, posterior pharynx, and into the esophageal hiatus. If more space is required to negotiate the turn in the posterior pharynx, it can be generated by further compressing the tongue anteriorly into the floor of the mouth while simultaneously opening the mandible.

The end point of blade insertion into the esophagus is achieved when the blade has been passed to its fullest extent. The proper application of cricoid pressure is not a deterrent to this maneuver. The angle where the laryngoscope handle meets the blade should be in apposition to the patient's teeth (Fig. 6.5). The importance of this relationship will be readily apparent when one begins the active, visual part of laryngoscopy and looks for the cords. When starting from this initial position, the cords are always proximal to the tip of the laryngoscope blade, never distal. In emergency laryngoscopy this is a significant advantage. If visual laryngoscopy is begun without passing the entire blade into the esophagus, the proximal position of the cords in relationship to the length of the blade cannot be assured, thus increasing the likelihood of not knowing what is initially visualized, and prompting the dreaded question, "Are the cords distal or more proximal?"

The second stage, or visual phase of laryngoscopy, will be more successful when the laryngoscopist assumes or creates a more comfortable intubating position that allows in-line visualization of the anatomic field. This can be accomplished by either raising the patient's stretcher or kneeling down on one knee to ensure that the airway is directly in the laryngoscopist's line of sight. Uncomfortable, contorted body positions unnecessarily complicate laryngoscopy. A tonsil suction (Yankauer) can be held in the laryngoscopist's right hand to remove any secretions, blood, emesis, or other debris that might be obscuring the visual field. Under constant direct vision the laryngoscope and blade are then withdrawn slowly in the same fashion as they were initially passed. Gentle listing pressure rather than strong muscle power is utilized as the laryngoscope is withdrawn. There should not be any rocking motion as this withdrawal is done (Fig. 6.2C). The maneuver is simply a continuous, even-pressured withdrawal of the laryngoscope until the cords are visualized, which almost always will be the first recognizable anatomic structure encountered (Fig. 6.6). The most common misperception that

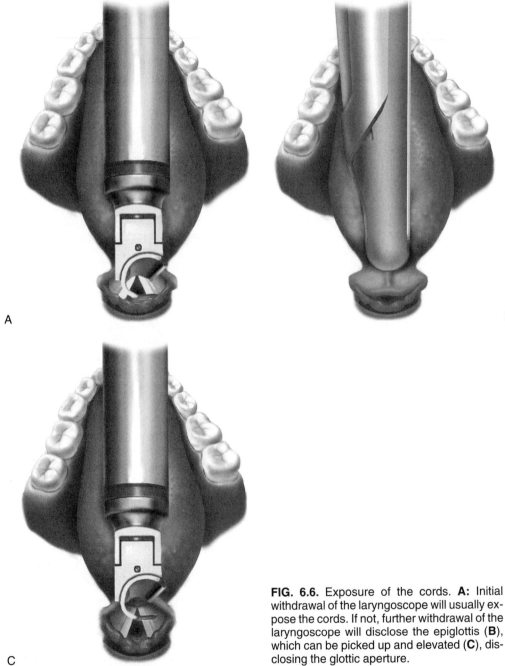

A

B

C

FIG. 6.6. Exposure of the cords. **A:** Initial withdrawal of the laryngoscope will usually expose the cords. If not, further withdrawal of the laryngoscope will disclose the epiglottis (**B**), which can be picked up and elevated (**C**), disclosing the glottic aperture.

occurs as this stage of laryngoscopy is performed is that the operator feels the blade has been withdrawn too far and the cords have been missed when, in fact, the cords still lie proximal to the current visual field and will be exposed momentarily. After the cords are identified, the ETT is passed through the glottic opening. Cormack and Lehane quantified the extent to which one is able to visualize the larynx, epiglottis, and upper airway during laryngoscopy (Fig. 6.7). Grades 1 and 2 are usually associated with low laryngoscopic failure rates, whereas grades 3 and 4 usually have high failure rates.

If the vocal cords lie anterior (the anterior airway) and are not adequately visualized or are simply not identified during initial laryngoscopy, continued steady withdrawal of the laryngoscope will disclose the epiglottis as it comes free from the compressing surface of the blade and drops into view. Once the epiglottis has been found, the constant anatomic relationship of the vocal cords to the epiglottis can be exploited. Under direct vision, the tip of the curved or straight blade is used to pick up and elevate the epiglottis, exposing the glottic aperture. If the laryngoscopic view is less than adequate for safe passage of the ETT (Fig. 6.3D), firm backward, upward, and rightward pressure on the thyroid cartilage with the laryngoscopist's free right hand (Fig. 6.3E) will most often improve the laryngeal view one full grade, producing maximal glottic exposure. (Fig. 6.3F). This maneuver, which is distinct from Sellick's maneuver, is called the "BURP" maneuver (*B*ackward-*U*pward-*R*ightward-*P*ressure). Once the vocal cords are exposed, a second assistant can maintain the BURP position, or the first assistant

Grade 1

Grade 2

Grade 3

Grade 4

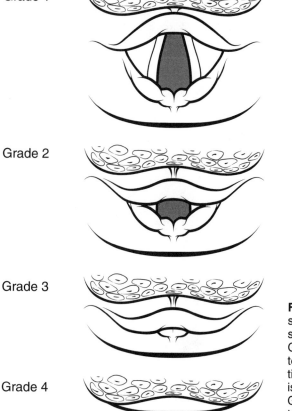

FIG. 6.7. Cormack-Lehane laryngoscopic grading system. Grade I is visualization of the entire glottic aperture. Grade II is visualization of just the arytenoid cartilages or the posterior portion of the glottic aperture. Grade III is visualization of only the epiglottis. Grade IV is visualization of only the tongue or the tongue and soft palate.

providing cricoid pressure with the right hand can use the left hand to perform the BURP maneuver, or the first assistant, without releasing cricoid pressure, can perform a combined Sellick-BURP with their right hand while the laryngoscopist intubates the trachea. Although it has been said that only a curved blade should be placed in the vallecula and only a straight blade should be used to manipulate the epiglottis, in reality, whichever blade can best manipulate the anatomic structures around the airway and provide the best view of the cords should be used.

Epiglottic identification is especially important in those infrequent situations in which the laryngoscopist is uncertain whether the exposed structure is the glottis or the esophagus. The glottic opening may be atypical in appearance, or there may have been traumatic changes in the appearance of the airway from previous prehospital or emergency department attempts at intubation. The esophageal hiatus or infrequent iatrogenic perilaryngeal tears can resemble the glottic aperture, especially when laryngeal exposure is limited. Absolute identification of the epiglottis in these and other doubtful cases will minimize the incidence of failed intubation. Occasionally, despite using the paraglossal technique of laryngoscopy, the laryngoscopist might be unable to identify either the cords or the epiglottis. Continued withdrawal of the laryngoscope will quickly disclose the base of the patient's tongue, a universally recognized structure. In this situation, gentle visual reinsertion of the blade should identify the epiglottis and help locate the glottic aperture.

Once the airway has been identified, it is important that the laryngoscopist not lose sight of the target, the glottic aperture. An assistant, who frequently is standing at the patient's right side applying Sellick's maneuver or Sellick-BURP, should retract the right side of the patient's mouth, allowing generous access to the oropharynx and, most important, providing room for unimpeded passage of the ETT (Fig. 6.8). The assistant should hand the ETT with an indwelling stylet to the laryngoscopist at the appropriate time. The ETT should be passed from the right side of the patient's mouth, initially toward the hard and soft palate, and should not be passed through the flange of the blade. If the ETT is passed down the flange of the blade, it can become entrapped, preventing

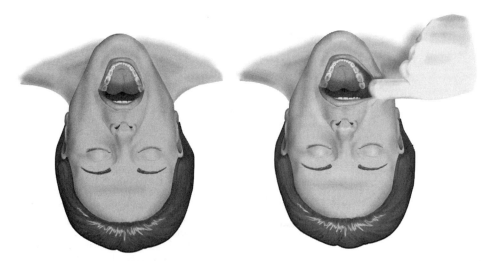

FIG. 6.8. Retraction of the corner of the mouth by an assistant's index finger will provide ample room for unobstructed passage of the ETT.

advancement or lacerating the balloon, necessitating reintubation. Additionally, entering from the right side of the patient's mouth prevents any obstruction or distraction of the laryngoscopist's view of the cords.

As the ETT is initially passed into the right side of the patient's mouth, the bevel of the tube should lie in a horizontal position. As the tube initially advances toward the palate and then curves upward toward the glottic opening, the bevel should be simultaneously rotated counterclockwise 90 degrees from the horizontal (widest) to the vertical (narrowest) plane to facilitate atraumatic passage through the cords (Fig. 6.9). This rotation will align the bevel in its thinnest, narrowest anatomic orientation. Following passage through the cords, the laryngoscope and the stylet are removed, the balloon is inflated, and the patient is appropriately oxygenated and ventilated. Proper tube position must then be confirmed by end-tidal carbon dioxide detection (gold standard), clinical assessment, and pulse oximetry response. When using a colorimetric end-tidal carbon dioxide detector, the color will quickly change from purple (poor) to yellow (yes). Any color other than yellow (e.g., tan) should be considered indeterminate and indicate probable esophageal intubation. Immediate steps must be taken to verify or correct tube position, including repeat laryngoscopy, immediate extubation with subsequent reoxygenation by bag and mask, and repeat laryngoscopy and intubation. Auscultation of the left supraclavicular area, left axilla, left chest, right chest, and epigastrium are additive to end-tidal carbon dioxide detection. The left side of the chest is preferentially auscultated first to confirm that a right mainstem intubation has not occurred. Chest x-ray is appropriate and is used primarily to assess for mainstem intubation and tube position within the trachea, not to determine whether tracheal intubation has occurred. "Fogging" (condensation) of the ETT during mechanical ventilation is a completely unreliable method of confirming tracheal intubation and should not be used.

III. Failed laryngoscopy

When tracheal intubation is unsuccessful, the patient should be reoxygenated and ventilated with a bag and mask. During this time, the laryngoscopist should systematically analyze the likely causes of the failure. It makes no sense to attempt a second laryngoscopy without changing something in the procedure to improve chances for success.

 • Is the patient in the optimum sniffing position for laryngoscopy and intubation? Is there something additional in terms of positioning that would improve the view of the vocal cords? If the patient's head is lying flat on the stretcher, the placement of a pillow, sheet,

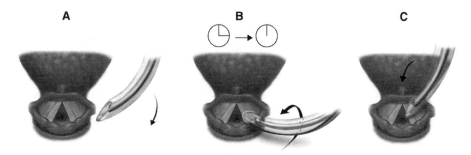

FIG. 6.9. The ETT is rotated 90 degrees counterclockwise (**B**) as it is passed through the cords, changing the initial horizontal (widest) axis of the bevel (**A**) to the vertical (narrowest) axis (**C**).

or blanket under the patient's head might improve the glottic view. If the patient was placed in the sniffing position initially and the larynx still appeared quite anterior, reducing the degree of head extension could be helpful. Additionally, it may help to elevate and *flex* the patient's head with the laryngoscopist's right hand (actually flex both the head and neck) while performing laryngoscopy to create a better view of an anterior airway.

- Would a different blade provide a better view? If the initial attempt at laryngoscopy is done with a curved blade, it may be advisable to change to a straight blade and vice versa. Alternatively, a larger blade of the same type might be helpful.
- Is the patient adequately paralyzed? Laryngoscopy may have been attempted too soon after administering succinylcholine. If the total time of paralysis has been such that the effect of succinylcholine is dissipating, then the administration of a second paralyzing dose of succinylcholine is advisable. Should this occur, atropine must be available to treat potential bradycardia that occasionally accompanies repeat dosing of succinylcholine.
- Was everything possible done to optimize the view of the cords? Would the BURP maneuver be helpful? Most often, BURP improves the laryngeal view by one full grade.
- Is a more experienced laryngoscopist available?

IV. Tips and pearls
- In patients with beards and moustaches, a water-soluble lubricant applied to the facial hair may improve mask seal.
- Edentulous or emaciated patients with concave cheeks may be difficult to ventilate with a bag and mask because of a poor mask seal. Replacement of dentures will facilitate bag-and-mask ventilation in the edentulous patient. Gauze sponges (4 × 4) may be fluffed and compressed, then inserted into the cheeks to create an improved mask seal. Care must be taken to avoid displacement of the gauze sponges into the airway, leading to upper-airway obstruction.
- "100% nonrebreather masks" generally deliver only 70% to 75% oxygen. If a chronic obstructive pulmonary disease (COPD) patient requires a reduced and measured concentration of oxygen, Venturi masks should be used.
- Nasal prongs deliver an oxygen concentration that can be approximated as (number of liters per minute) × 2 + 20. Thus 4L nasal prongs ought to approximate an inspired oxygen concentration of 28%. This is a very crude estimate and pulse oximetry should be followed closely. Also, if titration of oxygen is required (COPD), Venturi masks should be used.
- The right-sized (length) oropharyngeal airway in children is the one that spans the distance from the earlobe to the corner of the mouth. The Broselow-Luten tape provides this and additional information about equipment and drug dosing in pediatric airway management.

ADDITIONAL READING

Balk R. The technique of orotracheal intubation *J Crit Illness* 1997;12:316–323.
Benumof JL. Difficult laryngoscopy: obtaining the best view. *Can J Anaesth* 1994;41:361–365.
Bishop MJ, Bedford RF, Kil HK. Physiologic and pathophysiologic responses to intubation. In: Benumof JL, ed. *Airway management: principles and practice.* St Louis: Mosby, 1996:102–117.
Cormack RS, Lehane J. Difficult tracheal intubation in obstetrics *Anaesthesia* 1984;39:1105–1111.

Henderson J. The use of paraglossal straight blade laryngoscopy in difficult tracheal intubation. *Anaesthesia* 1997;52:552–560.

Takahata O, Kubota M, Mamiya K, et al. The efficacy of the "BURP" maneuver during a difficult laryngoscopy. *Anesth Analg* 1997;84:419–421.

Vender JS, Clemency MV. Nonintubation management of the airway: mask ventilation. In: Benumof JL, ed. *Airway management: principles and practice.* St Louis: Mosby, 1996:228–254.

7

RSI Using Competitive (Non-depolarizing) Neuromuscular Blocking Agents

John C. Sakles* and Ron M. Walls**

*Department of Emergency Medicine, University of Cincinnati College of Medicine, Cincinnati, Ohio; **Chairman, Department of Emergency Medicine, Brigham and Women's Hospital; Associate Professor of Medicine, Division of Emergency Medicine, Harvard Medical School, Boston, Massachusetts

I. Succinylcholine and RSI

From a pharmacokinetic standpoint succinylcholine (SCh) is the ideal neuromuscular blocking agent (NMBA) for rapid sequence intubation (RSI). When administered by rapid intravenous (IV) push, it reliably produces profound motor paralysis in 45 seconds and has a duration of action of less than 10 minutes. Adequate, spontaneous respirations return on average within 9 minutes of administration of SCh, a distinct advantage in the rare instance of a failed airway. Unfortunately, SCh has a number of adverse effects, which are described in great detail in Chapter 14. Adverse effects include fasciculations, hyperkalemia, increased intracranial pressure, and increased intraocular pressure. Rarely, SCh can result in malignant hyperthermia or anaphylaxis, although malignant hyperthermia has not yet been reported in an emergency department (ED) patient. Despite this formidable list of side effects, SCh in general is a fairly safe drug and can be used in the vast majority of patients undergoing RSI. From a clinical standpoint the most serious concern is SCh-induced hyperkalemia, which can occasionally precipitate fatal ventricular dysrhythmias. There are numerous case reports of patients suffering SCh-related cardiac arrests, presumably caused by hyperkalemia from the cellular release of potassium from depolarized myocytes.

II. SCh precautions and patient selection

There are essentially two groups of patients that are at risk of ventricular dysrhythmias secondary to SCh-induced hyperkalemia:

A. Patients with preexistent hyperkalemia in whom even a small rapid rise in serum potassium might result in ventricular irritability and dysrhythmias. These are usually patients with end-stage renal disease who have missed dialysis. Patients with a severe metabolic acidosis of any cause are at risk of having hyperkalemia due to cellular shifts in potassium. Some patients with severe, well-established rhabdomyolysis, such as the elderly patient who was "down" for an indeterminate amount of time, may also be at risk for hyperkalemia and exacerbation of this by succinylcholine.

B. Patients with certain medical or traumatic conditions that have an exaggerated release of potassium in response to SCh. Conditions associated with this exaggerated response are described in Chapter 14, including any form of muscular dystrophy, such as Duchenne's muscular dystrophy or pseudohypertrophic muscular dystrophy. Other conditions in which there is a functional denervation of muscle, such as subacute spinal cord injuries or strokes, also have been associated with excessive release of potassium. Patients with extensive burns more than 24 hours old or massive crush injuries at least several days old can also become extremely hyperkalemic in response to SCh. Patients with any of these clinical conditions should not be given SCh, as an intractable cardiac arrest may occur, despite timely recognition and appropriate treatment for hyperkalemia.

III. Nondepolarizing (competitive) NMBAs

When a patient has a clear contraindication to SCh, a nondepolarizing neuromuscular blocking agent must be used for RSI. Many nondepolarizing NMBAs are available, each with its own set of advantages and disadvantages. The biggest drawback to these competitive agents has been a longer onset of action and a longer duration of action than SCh. Rocuronium Bromide (Zemuron®) achieves intubating conditions uniformly in under 60 seconds and so had become the agent of choice for competitive RSI, supplanting vecuronium bromide for this purpose. However, a new, ultra-short acting competitive NMBA, rapacuronium bromide (Raplon®), approved by the FDA in 1999 offers the potential of more rapid attainment of paralysis and a shorter duration of action than either rocuronium or vecuronium. As a result, rapacuronium may offer the potential for large scale replacement of succinylcholine as the agent of choice for emergency RSI, but ED based studies are needed before this change will be indicated. From the RSI standpoint, familiarity with all three of these agents is necessary, although practitioners should choose just one upon which they will rely when competitive RSI is necessary.

A. Rapacuronium

Rapacuronium bromide (Raplon®, RAP) is a new, aminosteroid, competitive neuromuscular blocking agent, and is discussed in detail in chapter 14. When administered in a dose of 1.5 mg/kg with an appropriate induction agent, RAP achieves intubating level paralysis on a time line very similar to that of succinylcholine. Several studies have documented good to excellent intubation conditions for all patients by 60 seconds after administration, indistinguishable from succinylcholine. The duration of action of RAP is longer than for SCh, but neostigmine (0.05 mg/kg with glycopyrrolate 0.01 mg/kg) can be administered as early as two minutes after the RAP, resulting in dramatic reduction in duration of action. Used without neostigmine, clinical duration until recovery of adequate diaphragmatic ventilation with RAP 1.5 mg/kg is about 20 minutes, but with reversal, adequate spontaneous ventilation may be expected in approximately 10 minutes, and in a manner comparable to that of succinylcholine. Both 1.5 mg/kg and 2.5 mg/kg doses of RAP have been tested, and the 1.5 mg/kg dose appears to offer comparable intubating conditions with a significantly reduced duration of action, especially when neostigmine reversal is used. RAP has proven to be very hemodynamically stable.

Rapacuronium is provided in 5 and 10 ml vials and requires reconstitution with sterile water to produce a 20 mg/ml solution. It may be stored at room temperature.

B. Rocuronium

After rapacuronium, rocuronium (ROC) has the next most rapid onset of paralysis of all of the competitive (non-depolarizing) NMBAs. ROC has been quite widely used for competitive RSI in the ED. Administration of 1 mg/kg of ROC, along with a potent sedative/anesthetic agent such as etomidate, can result in satisfactory intubating conditions in less than 1 minute. At this dose, however, paralysis can last 40 to 60 minutes. This is a distinct disadvantage of ROC when compared to RAP. The increased duration of action is not a problem under most circumstances, but in the "can't intubate" situation, spontaneous respirations cannot be reestablished for at least 30 minutes, even if reversal agents are used. Additionally, use of ROC may complicate the ongoing evaluation of a patient with a head injury or status epilepticus, as serial neurologic exams will be unobtainable for a prolonged period (the duration of paralysis). Nonetheless, ROC is consistently effective, results in no change in serum potassium, is hemodynamically very safe, and has not been associated with malignant hyperthermia. It comes in liquid form in 50-mg vials, which should be kept refrigerated. At room temperature it has a shelf life of 30 days. Note that the "priming principle," as explained later for vecuronium (VEC), is *not* effective or necessary with ROC.

C. Vecuronium

Vecuronium is another nondepolarizing NMBA that has been used in EDs for several years. Structurally, it is an analog of ROC and shares many of its advantageous properties, such as minimal side effects. Unfortunately, at the standard dose of 0.1 mg/kg the onset of paralysis can be as long as 2 to 3 minutes when given by rapid IV push. Invariably, this delay necessitates assisted bag-and-mask ventilation (BMV) as patients often desaturate before intubating level paralysis is established. This is not the ideal situation in a patient with a full stomach who is at risk of aspiration. Additionally, the duration of action of VEC is much longer than that of SCh, ROC, or RAP, resulting in paralysis for 30 to 40 minutes. VEC comes as a powder in 10-mg vials that must be reconstituted with saline prior to its use.

There are two key strategies to hasten VEC's onset of action. First, a very large dose of VEC can be administered. Studies have shown that a dose that is three times the normal intubating dose (i.e., 0.3 mg/kg) can result in adequate intubating conditions in approximately 60 to 90 seconds. Using these large doses of VEC, however, will also considerably increase the duration of paralysis to upward of 100 minutes. The other method that has been demonstrated to hasten the onset of VEC is to employ a technique known as the "priming principle." This method uses a very small dose of VEC (usually one-tenth of the intubating dose, or 0.01 mg/kg), given intravenously 2 to 3 minutes prior to the administration of an increased intubating dose of 0.15 mg/kg. This technique can also reduce the onset of paralysis to approximately 60 to 90 seconds. One must use caution when using this method, as the small initial dose can infrequently result in the complete cessation of respiratory effort in the compromised patient. Consequently, one must be prepared to intubate the patient immediately after giving the priming dose of VEC. Side effects are few, and there are no clinically significant changes in blood pressure with VEC. There is no cellular release of potassium with VEC, RAP, or ROC and thus no hyperkalemia. In general, using 1.5 mg/kg of RAP, 1.0 mg/kg of ROC, or 0.3 mg/kg of VEC, eliminates the need to use the priming principle in the ED.

IV. The timing principle

When using SCh and an anesthetic agent such as etomidate, the onset times are so similar that the two drugs are typically administered simultaneously. Thus the patient becomes paralyzed as consciousness is lost. When using VEC or ROC, the onset of paralysis will take somewhat longer than with SCh. Thus if the NMBA and anesthetic agent are given simultaneously, the patient may become unconscious, with depressed respirations; be unable to protect his or her airway; but not have the level of neuromuscular blockade that will permit intubation. It thus may be advantageous to *administer the nondepolarizing NMBA first,* follow the patient closely, and then when first signs of the onset of weakness become apparent, administer the anesthetic agent. In this fashion paralysis and unconsciousness will occur at the same time. This technique is referred to in the literature as the "timing principle," which is distinct from the "priming principle" described earlier, and has been used successfully with both ROC and VEC. There is no evidence that the timing approach is superior to the bolus and priming approaches outlined above, and in any case, no such modification of technique is necessary when RAP 1.5 mg/kg is used. There is probably no need to consider using the timing principle in the ED with ROC either.

A. RSI using competitive agents

1. Rapacuronium
  a. Preparation
  b. Preoxygenation
  c. Pretreatment
  - As indicated by patient condition
  - "Defasciculation" not required

  d. Paralysis with induction
  - Etomidate 0.3 mg/kg IV
  - Rapacuronium 1.5 mg/kg IV

  e. Protection and positioning
  f. Placement with proof
  - At 45 seconds

2. Rocuronium
  a. Preparation
  b. Preoxygenation
  c. Pretreatment
  - As indicated by patient condition
  - "Defasciculation" not required

  d. Paralysis with induction
  - Etomidate 0.3 mg/kg IV
  - Rocuronium 1.0 mg/kg IV

  e. Protection and positioning
  f. Placement with proof
  - At 45 seconds

  g. Postintubation management

3. Vecuronium 0.3 mg/kg dose
  a. Preparation
  b. Preoxygenation
  c. Pretreatment
  - As indicated by patient condition
  - "Defasciculation" not required

  d. Paralysis with induction
  - Etomidate 0.3 mg/kg IV
  - Vecuronium 0.3 mg/kg IV

  e. Protection and positioning
  f. Placement with proof
  - At 60 seconds

  g. Postintubation management

4. Vecuronium using the priming principle
  a. Preparation
  b. Preoxygenation
  c. Pretreatment
  - As indicated by patient condition
  - Vecuronium 0.01 mg/kg IV

  d. Paralysis with induction
  - Etomidate 0.3 mg/kg IV
  - Vecuronium 0.15 mg/kg IV
  e. Protection and positioning
  f. Placement with proof
  - At 60 seconds
  g. Postintubation management

ADDITIONAL READING

Agoston S. Onset time and evaluation of intubating conditions: rocuronium in perspective. *Eur J Anaesthesiol* 1995;11[Suppl]:31–37.

Alastair JJ, Wood MD. New neuromuscular blocking drugs. *N Engl J Med* 1995;332:1691–1699.

Culling RC, Middaugh RE, Menk EJ. Rapid tracheal intubation with vecuronium: the timing principle. *J Clin Anesth* 1989;1:422–425.

DeMey JC, Debrock M, Rolly G. Evaluation of the onset and intubation conditions of rocuronium bromide. *Eur J Anaesthesiol* 1994;9[Suppl]:37–40.

Fisher DM, Kahwaji R, Bevan D, et al. Factors affecting the pharmacokinetic characteristics of rapacuronium. *Anesthesiology* 1999;90:993–1000.

Fleming NW, Chung F, Glass PS, et al. Comparison of the intubation conditions provided by rapacuronium (ORG9487) or succinylcholine in humans during anesthesia with fentanyl and propofol. *Anesthesiology* 1999;91:1311–1317.

Kirkegaard-Nielsen H, Caldwell JE, Berry PD. Rapid tracheal intubation with rocuronium: a probability approach to determining dose. *Anesthesiology* 1999;91:131–136.

Larach MG, Rosenberg H, Gronert GA, et al. Hyperkalemic cardiac arrest during anesthesia in infants and children with occult myopathies. *Clin Pediatr* 1997;36:9–16.

Magorian T, Flannery KB, Miller RD. Comparison of rocuronium, succinylcholine, and vecuronium for rapid sequence induction of anesthesia in adult patients. *Anesthesiology* 1993;79:913–918.

Mazurek AJ, Rae B, Hann S, Kim JI, Castro B, Cote CJ. Rocuronium versus succinylcholine: are they equally effective during rapid-sequence induction of anasthesia? *Anesthesia* 1998;87:1259–1262.

Nelson JM, Morell RC, Butterworth JF 4th. Rocuronium versus succinylcholine for rapid-sequence induction using a variation of the timing principle. *J Clin Anesth* 1997;9:317–320.

Onrust SV, Foster RH. Rapacuronium bromide: a review of its use in anaesthetic practice. *Drugs* 1999;58:887–918.

Purdy R, Bevan DR, Donati F, Lichtor JL. Early reversal of rapacuronium with neostigmine. *Anesthesiology* 1999;91:51–57.

Robertson EN, Hull JM, Verbeek AM, et al. A comparison of rocuronium and vecuronium: the pharmacodynamic, cardiovascular and intra-ocular effects. *Eur J Anaesth* 1994;9[Suppl]:116–121.

Rubin MA, Sadovnikoff N. Neuromuscular blocking agents in the emergency department. *J Emerg Med* 1996;14:193–199.

Schwarz SI, Ilias W, Lackner F, et al. Rapid tracheal intubation with vecuronium: the priming principle. *Anesthesiology* 1985;62:388–391.

Weiss JH, Gratz I, Goldberg ME, et al. Double-blind comparison of two doses of rocuronium and succinylcholine for rapid-sequence intubation. *J Clin Anesth* 1997;9:379–382.

8

Awake Intubation Techniques

Ron M. Walls* and Robert C. Luten†

*Chairman, Department of Emergency Medicine, Brigham and Women's Hospital,
Associate Professor of Medicine, Division of Emergency Medicine, Harvard Medical School,
Boston, Massachusetts; †Professor of Emergency Medicine and Pediatrics,
University of Florida, Jacksonville, Florida

Awake intubation techniques comprise all techniques in which consciousness is intentionally maintained during the intubation. This is to be distinguished from the practice of administering sedating drugs in lieu of neuromuscular blocking agents to facilitate unconscious intubation. The three most common of these awake techniques are blind nasotracheal intubation, awake oral intubation, and fiberoptic intubation.

I. Blind nasotracheal intubation

Although blind nasotracheal intubation (NTI) was very widely used in emergency departments in the past, it is rapidly being supplanted by superior techniques of oral intubation with neuromuscular blockade, even in the prehospital setting. In general, nasotracheal intubation has a number of very serious drawbacks, and very few advantages (if any) over the other techniques that are readily available. Principally, the nasotracheal technique takes longer, has a higher failure rate, has a higher complication rate, and requires smaller tube sizes than rapid sequence oral intubation.

A. Indications and contraindications

As clinicians become more facile and comfortable with neuromuscular blockade and a variety of other approaches, it is likely that the one remaining indication for NTI may be the patient with a difficult airway who is breathing spontaneously, and for whom rapid sequence intubation (RSI) may not be advisable (Chapter 3). NTI is achieved by listening to the patient's spontaneous respirations through the tube and so should not be considered if the patient is apneic. It is contraindicated in combative patients; in those with anatomically disturbed airways; in those with neck hematomas; in cases of increased intracranial pressure; in the context of severe facial trauma, upper airway infection, obstruction, or abscess; and in the presence of coagulopathy. It should be performed with great reservation on any patient who needs rapid intubation, because, despite optimistic claims to the contrary, intubation usually requires several minutes to complete using this technique. Therefore it is a poor choice for patients with respiratory failure, such as the asthmatic patient in extremis, who cannot be oxygenated during the protracted intubation attempt. In addition, one of the primary indications for nasotracheal intubation in the past, the multiply injured patient with potential cervical spine injury, has been discarded, and oral rapid sequence intubation with in-line stabilization is now the recommended route (see Chapter 18).

B. The technique of NTI is as follows:

   1. Preoxygenate the patient with 100% oxygen for several minutes if possible. Try to avoid bagging with positive pressure if spontaneous ventilation is adequate.

   2. Choose the nostril to be used. Inspect the interior of the nares, with particular reference to the septum and turbinates. It may help to occlude each nostril in turn and listen to the flow of air through the orifices. If there appears no clear favorite, the right naris should be selected, as it better facilitates passage of the tube with the bevel out (see later).

   3. Place two or three drops of 0.5% neosynephrine or oxymetazoline nasal solution in each nostril. This will vasoconstrict the nasal mucosa and make tube passage easier. The incidence of epistaxis may also be reduced. It may also be helpful to soak two or three cotton-tipped applicators in the neosynephrine solution and place them gently fully into the naris until the tip touches the nasopharynx. This provides vasoconstriction at the area that is often most difficult to negotiate blindly with the endotracheal tube. Insertion of a 4% cocaine pack or instillation of 2% lidocaine jelly will provide anesthesia for the nose. The oral cavity can be sprayed with 4% lidocaine or a similar spray, and, if desired, the pharynx may be anesthetized similarly. An alternative is to provide a solution of 4 ml of 4% lidocaine with 1 ml of 0.5% neosynephrine by aerosol. This takes approximately 5 to 10 minutes but provides excellent anesthesia, and is well tolerated. Still another suggested method involves insertion of an absorbent nasal tampon (as is used for epistaxis) and application of several milliliters of 2% lidocaine with 1:100,000 epinephrine. Cricothyroid puncture with instillation of 5 to 10 ml of 1% to 2% lidocaine is often advocated. This technique is reasonably simple and effective but usually produces coughing, perhaps an undesirable result. Complete anesthesia of the glottis may not be desirable in all cases. Advancing the tube during a cough sometimes allows immediate intubation of an otherwise elusive trachea. If the patient is awake, explain the procedure. This is a crucial step that is often neglected. If the patient becomes combative during the intubation, the attempt must cease, as epistaxis, turbinate damage, or even pharyngeal perforation may ensue. A brief, reassuring explanation of the procedure and its necessity may avert this undesirable situation.

   4. Lubricate the tube and the nostril. The use of 2% lidocaine jelly is often advocated, but it is unlikely that the brief contact between the jelly and the nasal mucosa results in anesthesia. However, the jelly is an adequate lubricant and is not harmful, so it is a reasonable choice.

   5. Select the appropriate size of ETT. In general, the tube should be the largest one that will fit through the nostril without inducing significant trauma. In most patients, a tube with an internal diameter (ID) of 6.0 to 7.5 cm will be chosen. If a difficult intubation is anticipated, a tube one size smaller than usual should be chosen. A smaller tube will fit through a difficult or tight space better than a larger tube. Test the ETT cuff for leaks.

   6. It is probably easiest for a right-handed person to intubate from the patient's left side. This allows the right hand to be used for the intubation, while the left hand applies cricoid pressure and provides feedback to the right hand. By leaning slightly forward between the two hands, the operator can listen to the breath sounds and guide the tube into place. Alternatively, a position immediately above the patient's head may be chosen. The patient may be placed in any comfortable position. The sitting position may be better, as it moves the tongue forward. Positioning the head as for oral intubation is worthwhile, however. The so-called sniffing position, with the neck flexed on the body and the head extended on the neck, optimizes the alignment of the mouth and pharynx with the vocal cords and trachea. A small towel may be placed behind the patient's occiput to help maintain this relationship.

7. Gently insert the tube into the nostril. For consistency, the remainder of this discussion will assume a right naris intubation by a right-handed operator. The tube should be turned so that the leading edge of the bevel is "out" (i.e., away from the septum). This will minimize the chances of septum injury and epistaxis. This also positions the tube with the natural curve upward, which facilitates the slightly upward direction of the distal tip of the tube to clear the lower turbinate. Once the tip of the tube is past the inferior turbinate, it should be directed caudad at approximately a 10-degree angle to follow the gently downsloping floor of the nose. This entire process should be done very slowly and with meticulous care. Once the nose is successfully intubated, further induction of epistaxis is unlikely. When the tip of the tube approaches the posterior pharynx, resistance will often be felt. At this point, rotate the proximal end of the tube approximately one-fourth of a turn toward the left nostril. This will place the short side of the bevel in the superior position and will facilitate "turning the corner" from the nose into the nasopharynx. Once the nasopharynx is successfully entered, restore the tube to the neutral (sagittal) position and proceed.

8. The tube should now be advanced until the breath sounds are best heard through it (usually approximately 3 to 5 cm). At this point, the distal tip of the tube is positioned immediately above the vocal cords. This process may be facilitated by occluding the opposite naris and closing the mouth.

9. Simultaneous with an inspiratory effort by the patient, advance the tube gently but firmly 3 to 4 cm while applying cricoid pressure with the left hand. The vocal cords abduct during inspiration and are most widely separated at this time.

10. When the tube is advanced, one of three things will happen. If the trachea is entered, a series of long, wheezy coughs will usually emanate from the patient. Inflation of the cuff and a few ventilations with an end-tidal carbon dioxide detector will confirm intratracheal placement. If the trachea is not entered, the tube either will slide easily down the esophagus or will come to an abrupt halt as it tries to pass anterior to the vocal cords or abuts against the anterior wall of the larynx. In the former case, the patient will not cough and ventilation through the tube will be better heard over the stomach than over the lungs. If the tube has passed down the esophagus, it is necessary to bring the distal tip of the tube further anteriorly. Withdraw the tube until the breath sounds are well heard again. Then extend the patient's head slightly and try again. If the intubation is being performed on a patient with possible cervical spine trauma, movement is impossible, in which case the intubation should be reattempted without any change in patient position. Use of the "Endotrol" tube, which has a ringlike apparatus connected to the distal end to allow anterior deflection of the tip of the tube, may be extremely helpful in such cases. If the tube has met with a "dead end," it is anterior to the cords or abutted against the anterior wall of the trachea. It may be possible to ascertain by palpation with the left hand whether the tube is off to the left, off to the right, or anterior in the midline. If the tube is truly anterior, slight withdrawal of the tube until breath sounds are well heard followed by slight flexion of the head should facilitate passage. This is a common pitfall. When a first attempt fails, the operator often continues to further extend the neck in an attempt to succeed, each extension making the situation anatomically more impossible. If it is felt that the tube

is off to the left or right in addition to being anterior, withdraw the tube, flex the head slightly, and turn the head slightly in the direction that the distal tip of the tube was off the midline. That is, if the distal tip of the tube is off to the right, turn the head to the right. The naris will lead the proximal end of the tube to the right, and the distal end will swing to the left, the desired corrective direction. Alternatively, the proximal end of the ETT may be rotated to the side where the distal end was detected to achieve this effect.

11. Inflate the cuff and confirm position with end-tidal carbon dioxide. A chest radiograph should also be obtained. If the presence of the tube or inflation of the cuff leads to prolonged coughing by the patient, administer 2 ml of 2% lidocaine solution through the ETT. This will often dramatically improve tube tolerance in seconds.

12. Only 60% to 70% of intubations will succeed on the first attempt. The "blind" nature of the procedure requires adjustment and attention to feedback. If the intubation is proving extremely difficult, consider:
    - Passing a fiberoptic laryngoscope or bronchoscope through the tube into the trachea (Chapter 10).
    - Passing a suction catheter or nasogastric tube through the ETT into the trachea. The suction catheter may enter the trachea more easily, and once in, will often guide the previously stubborn tube to its desired position.
    - Using the Endotrol tube.
    - Changing to a new tube, perhaps one that is 0.5 to 1.0 mm ID smaller. The tube often becomes warm and soft during the intubation attempt and is no longer capable of being appropriately manipulated.
    - Using a laryngoscope and Magill forceps. This may require conditions that are not present (i.e., the ability to insert a laryngoscope into the mouth and visualize the vocal cords).
    - Grasping the tongue with a piece of gauze and pulling it forward or sitting the patient up (if possible). This may improve the angle at the back of the tongue.
    - Abandoning the attempt. Prolonged attempts are associated with hypoxemia and glottic edema caused by local trauma. Either of these situations can worsen the situation substantially. Repeated attempts are not significantly more successful than the first. In 10 to 20% of cases, NTI will simply not be possible.
    - In an unconscious patient, the nasal passage may be dilated with a nasopharyngeal airway or a gloved small finger.

II. Awake oral intubation

When the patient who requires intubation also has a condition that will render both intubation and bag valve mask ventilation difficult, consideration should be given to performing an awake oral intubation. In this technique, a sedative agent is administered, liberal airway anesthesia is provided, and the patient is intubated orally, with a laryngoscope, "awake." In this context, *awake* means that the patient can follow simple instructions, provide feedback to the operator, and respond to what is happening. The classic context for awake intubation is the patient with distorted upper-airway anatomy, such as that resulting from blunt or penetrating anterior neck trauma, who requires intubation. Although the anatomy may appear normal, it may be distorted to the point that initial attempts at laryngoscopy and intubation will be unsuccessful. Positive-pressure ventilation using a bag and mask may result in the expulsion of large amounts of air into the neck through the airway injury, making the ventilation ineffective and exacerbating the situation. In this type of circumstance, one would like to ensure that laryngoscopy will permit visualization of the vocal cords prior to the initiation of an irreversible step, such as neuromuscular blockade. A recommended approach is as follows:

1. **Prepare the patient.** Ensure that the patient is well oxygenated and that the procedure has been explained to the greatest extent possible to alleviate fear and facilitate cooperation. Assemble all necessary equipment.

2. **Anesthetize the airway.** There are two common approaches. If time is not an issue, a solution of 4% lidocaine (4 ml) and 0.5% neosynephrine (1 ml) or 2% lidocaine (5 ml) + 2% lidocaine with 1:100,000 epinephrine (5 ml) can be nebulized using a standard respiratory nebulizer. Good airway anesthesia will be achieved in about 10 minutes. Alternatively, the standard method is to spray the mouth, tongue, oropharynx, and larynx with lidocaine spray using a laryngeal spray device. This requires a little patience and compassion but is extremely effective.

3. **Sedate the patient.** This is usually done just before, or at the same time as, the topical anesthesia, depending on the method and agents chosen. A good choice would be 1 to 2 mg of midazolam, accompanied by 50 to 100 mcg of fentanyl (for analgesia) if desired. Both of these drugs require 3 to 5 minutes to demonstrate peak effects, so the timing of the sedation, anesthesia, and intubation is important. Titration is necessary.

4. **Perform the laryngoscopy.** Talk to the patient, depending on the level of consciousness; gently advance the laryngoscope to where the cords can be visualized. The patient should be obtunded but breathing spontaneously throughout. At this point, the ETT can be inserted, or more potent agents, such as neuromuscular blocking agents and additional sedation, can be administered, followed by intubation, if desired. Visualization of the cords with laryngoscopy demonstrates the adequacy of the approach and may permit the administration of neuromuscular blocking agents if this is considered desirable. Whether to intubate immediately or defer for later and a controlled RSI will depend on the potential for progressively increased airway difficulty. One might elect to immediately intubate an airway burn or anaphylaxis with progressive swelling, whereas a patient with a stable anatomic picture, being intubated for another reason such as head injury, might be better served by deferring momentarily for a controlled RSI.

5. **Consider the need for additional sedation.** Also, as with all intubations in the emergency department, independent confirmation of tube placement and a chest radiograph are mandatory.

6. The identical sequence can be used to facilitate awake fiberoptic intubation (see Chapter 10).

ADDITIONAL READING

Bourke DL, Katz J, Tonneson A. Nebulized anesthesia for awake intubation. *Anesthesiology* 1985;63:690–692.

Dronen SC, Merigian KS, Hedges JR, et al. A comparison of blind nasotracheal and succinylcholine-assisted intubation in the poisoned patient. *Ann Emerg Med* 1987;16:650–652.

Rhec KJ, O'Malley BJ. Neuromuscular blockade assisted oral intubation vs. nasotracheal intubation in prehospital care of injured patients. *Ann Emerg Med* 1994;28:37.

Rourke DL, Katz J, Tonneson A. Nebulized anesthesia for awake intubation. *Anesthesiology* 1985;83:690–692.

Sanchez A, Trivedi N, Morrison P. Preparation of the patient for awake intubation. In: Benumof JL, ed. *Airway management: principles and practice.* St Louis: Mosby, 1996:159–182.

Tintanelli JE, Caffey J. Complications of nasotracheal intubation. *Am J Emerg Med* 1981;10:142.

9

Special Devices and Techniques for Managing the Difficult or Failed Airway

Michael F. Murphy

Departments of Emergency Medicine and Anaesthesiology,
Queen Elizabeth II Health Sciences Centre, Dalhousie University, Halifax, Nova Scotia

While direct-vision laryngoscopy and intubation has been proven over the years to be reliable and relatively easy, the accurate and prompt placement of an endotracheal tube (ETT) remains a major challenge in some patients, even in the hands of experienced laryngoscopists. It has been estimated that between 1% and 3% of patients present with difficult airways, leading to difficult endotracheal intubation under direct vision using a laryngoscope. In fact, it is impossible to intubate some patients with this technique, emphasizing the key role of cricothyrotomy in emergency airway management. The National Emergency Airway Registry reported a 1% incidence of cricothyrotomy among 1,288 emergency department (ED) patients in 11 centers.

ETTs can be guided into place nonsurgically in the following ways:

- Under direct vision (via a laryngoscope, bronchoscope, etc.)
- With an indirect indicator, such as listening to and feeling air movement in nasal intubation, transillumination of light in the neck with lighted stylets and bronchoscopes, and tactile digital intubation
- Blindly, without an indicator

Many devices and techniques designed to rescue the patient in the event of a failed intubation have been described. This chapter will describe the lighted stylet intubation device and technique as well as the techniques of retrograde and digital intubation, that may be techniques usually indicated when intubation has failed, though it is still possible to ventilate the patient (i.e., the "*can't* intubate, *can* ventilate" situation).

It will also discuss the use of the laryngeal mask airway (LMA) and the esophageal tracheal Combitube, rescue devices for the patient who cannot be intubated *or* ventilated ("*can't* intubate, *can't* ventilate") and on whom cricothyrotomy cannot be performed immediately.

Neither of these latter two devices constitutes definitive airway management, defined as a device that:

- Facilitates the maintenance of normal blood gas tensions.
- Protects the airway from aspiration.
- Allows the management of pulmonary secretions (pulmonary "toilette").

The LMA and Combitube are temporizing measures only in emergency airway management, buying time until definitive control is achieved. In addition, they are very stimulating to place and maintain; thus patients who are eligible for them must be deeply sedated, obtunded, or paralyzed.

I. Lighted-stylet intubation

Lighted-stylet intubation is of use in those situations where conventional laryngoscopy has failed to provide visualization of the larynx sufficient to allow direct-vision laryngoscopy and intubation. In other words, the conventional method laryngoscopic technique has failed and another technique is required. Ventilation and oxygenation must be possible to allow time for the use of the lightwand (i.e., "cannot intubate, can oxygenate"), and the risk of regurgitation and aspiration must be minimized.

A. Definition

This light-guided intubation technique relies on the transillumination of the soft tissues of the neck to indicate correct tube positioning. It was first used in 1959 by Yamamura and colleagues in Japan for blind nasal intubation. This technique takes advantage of the anterior location of the trachea, relative to the esophagus. With the light bulb of a lightwand placed at the tip of the ETT, a well-defined circumscribed glow can readily be seen in the anterior neck area when the tip of the tube enters the glottic opening and trachea. However, if the tip of the tube is in the esophagus, the light glow is diffuse and not easily seen. Although the light-guided intubation technique had shown some promise, it was not widely used until the 1970s, following the introduction of the Flexilum (Concept Corporation, Clearwater, FL). The Tubestat (Concept Corporation, Clearwater, FL) was developed in the early 1980s, following minor refinements of the original Flexilum design. Despite these improvements, difficulties persisted with the use of these devices. A lightwand device from Vital Signs (Vital Light) has recently been introduced. It has the advantage of a bright light and low cost. A device known as the Trachlight (Laerdal Medical Corp., Armonk, NY) has incorporated many modifications to improve flexibility to allow oral and nasal intubation. The remainder of the discussion will refer to the Trachlight device, or "lightwand."

B. Indications and contraindications

As with all procedures, facility with the device to allow predictable success rates requires practice in a controlled setting. It has been demonstrated that this technique is easier to teach and the skill is easier to maintain than is true with conventional laryngoscopy. It also produces less airway trauma and physiologic disturbance than conventional laryngoscopy. However, the vast majority of emergency physicians will continue to be more skillful with the laryngoscope than with the lightwand. This device is likely to serve as a backup device to be tried when orotracheal intubation by other techniques is impossible (e.g., Temperomandibular Joint (TMJ) ankylosis, limitation of C-spine mobility) because of inability to visualize the glottis, and bag-and-mask ventilation is adequate. The device can be used to facilitate nasotracheal as well as orotracheal intubation.

The "can't intubate, can't oxygenate" situation is a relative contraindication because of the time required, unless the operator has considerable skill and experience with the device. As with conventional intubation techniques, this technique requires moderate to substantial sedation or obtundation. Airway obstruction suspected to be due to laryngeal lesions should only be managed by direct-vision techniques; this technique is therefore contraindicated in this situation.

C. Technique

The Trachlight device consists of two parts: a reusable handle and a disposable wand. The power control circuitry and batteries are encased within the handle. The Trachlight requires three AAA alkaline batteries, which can be changed by opening the cover on the handle. A female connector with a locking lever located on the front of the handle accepts and secures the standard 7-mm male connector of ETTs. The wand consists of a durable, flexible plastic tube with a bright light bulb at one end. The light bulb is sufficiently bright to permit transillumination and intubation under ambient light in most cases. Affixed to the other end of the wand is a rigid plastic connector with a release arm, which fastens the wand onto the top surface of the handle. This connector can be adjusted and glided along the handle to accommodate ETTs of different lengths. Enclosed within the plastic tube of the wand is a rigid, but malleable, retractable stylet. During intubation, the ETT and the wand become pliable when the rigid stylet is retracted. This facilitates the advancement of the tube into the trachea.

1. *Preparation.* To ensure easy retraction during intubation, the internal rigid stylet of the wand should be well lubricated. Similarly, the external wall of the wand should be lubricated with a water-soluble lubricant. With the Trachlight in place, the ETT should be bent just proximal to the endotracheal cuff, into a right angle, mimicking the shape of a "field hockey stick." The tip of the ETT should also be lubricated with a water-soluble lubricant.

2. *Positioning.* With the intubator standing at the head of the patient, the neck is bared to allow maximal visualization of the anterior neck of the patient during intubation. The technique can also be performed from the side of the patient. Usually, the patient's head and neck are placed in a neutral position, though it may be necessary to extend the head slightly to optimize visualization. In obese patients or patients with an extremely short neck, placing a pillow under the shoulder and neck may be helpful.

3. *Ambient lighting.* In general, patients can be intubated easily under ambient lighting conditions. Dimming the light or shading the neck to optimize visualization of the transilluminated glow may be necessary in those with thick, fat, or pigmented necks.

4. *Technique of intubation.* With the patient lying supine, the lower alveolar ridge and mentum are grasped and lifted upward using the intubator's nondominant hand. This lifts the tongue and epiglottis upward to facilitate the intubation. The nondominant hand must be kept close to the lower lip to ensure an unobstructed path in the midline for the lightwand. The device is then switched on and the ETT/lightwand combination (ETT-LW) is inserted into the oropharynx and positioned in the midline. The ETT-LW is then advanced gently to the right pyriform recess and the intensity of the transilluminated glow through the neck is noted. The intensity of this glow will approximate that found in the midline with successful placement of the device in the trachea. The device is then rocked back and forth in the midline in an imaginary arc that is anticipated to allow successful placement of the ETT-LW in the glottis. The jaw lift helps to elevate the epiglottis and enhance the passage of the ETT-LW under the epiglottis into the airway. When the tip of ETT-LW enters the glottic opening, a well-defined circumscribed glow can be seen at the anterior neck slightly below the laryngeal prominence. Retracting the rigid stylet 5-10 cm makes the ETT-LW more pliable and facilitates its advance into the trachea. The tip of the ETT is advanced until the glow appears in the sternal notch. At this point, the tip of the ETT is midway between the vocal cords and carina.

D. Success rates and complications

Success rates in the hands of experienced users are consistent with or exceed those associated with conventional laryngoscopy. Limited experience with this device has not identified isolated or persistent complications.

E. Tips and pearls
- Maintain gentle upward traction on the mandible.
- Rock the ETT-LW gently back and forth in the midline; force is not necessary.
- Rotate the ETT-LW tip from side to side in the hypopharynx and identify the direction of maximum transillumination. Then rock forward in that direction.
- Place the bend in the ETT-LW just proximal to the balloon of the ETT in normal individuals; more proximally in those with long necks; more distally in those with short necks. Make a good right angle bend.

II. Retrograde intubation

As with lightwand intubation, retrograde intubation does require time to be performed successfully and is most appropriately applied in the "can't intubate, can oxygenate" scenario.

A. Definition

Retrograde intubation involves a puncture of the cricothyroid membrane and the threading of a wire retrogradely through the vocal cords into the mouth or nose. This wire is then used to guide an ETT through the glottis.

B. Indications and contraindications

This technique should be considered:
- If C-spine motion is to be avoided and difficulty is anticipated with conventional techniques;
- As an alternative if intubation is anticipated to be difficult or impossible;
- In cases of failed intubation where bag-and-mask ventilation is adequate and time is available.

This technique should be avoided if the cricoid puncture is to be performed through an infected area. Infectious and neoplastic laryngeal lesions constitute relative contraindications to any nondirect visualization technique.

C. Technique

Commercially available, self-contained retrograde intubation kits are available on the market and facilitate the procedure. Continuous oxygen delivery via nasal prongs should be continued throughout the procedure in the spontaneously breathing patient.

1. The patient's neck is extended slightly if possible.
2. Palpate the cricothyroid membrane and infiltrate local anesthetic if required.
3. Puncture the membrane with a needle of sufficient caliber to accommodate the guidewire, stopping when air is aspirated, and direct it cephalad. Some have recommended the injection of lidocaine at this juncture, though it must be recognized that this may precipitate coughing and risk injury to airway and other nearby structures.
4. Thread the wire through the needle, with the soft J end leading, guiding the wire cephalad through the cords into the oropharynx.
5. Use a laryngoscope to visualize the wire in the oropharynx and use Magill forceps to pick up the wire and pull it out through the mouth. (In those unusual circumstances where nasotracheal intubation is contemplated, one can attempt to guide the wire retrogradely through the nose, though it is easier and quicker to use a catheter or ETT inserted through the nose to drag or guide the wire back through the nose.)
6. Pass the wire through the Murphy eye (outside to inside) and out the proximal end of the ETT. Put tension on either end of wire and slide ETT into place through the glottic opening. Techniques utilizing bronchoscopes and rigid guides passed over the retrograde wire designed to stiffen the system and enhance successful passage of the ETT have been described.
7. Once the ETT is at the level of the cricoid and meets resistance from the wire, cut the wire at the skin and advance the ETT into the trachea.
8. Pull the wire out through the proximal end of the ETT.

D. Success rates and complications

High success rates are reported in the hands of individuals experienced in the technique. The time required to perform the technique renders it ill suited to the failed-airway situation, where one is able neither to intubate nor to oxygenate.

Complications, although not reported for this specific procedure, are likely to be consistent with those from cricothyroid membrane puncture and include:

- Tracheal laceration
- Infection, including soft-tissue neck infections and mediastinitis
- Injuries to the larynx and vocal apparatus, including recurrent nerve damage

E. Tips and pearls

If a kit system is not being used, a Tuohy needle, usually used to insert epidural catheters, is a good choice, because the needle is designed to allow the wire to be more easily directed cephalad.

III. Digital intubation

A. Definition

Digital intubation is a tactile intubation technique in which the intubator uses his or her fingers to direct an ETT into the larynx. The technique has gained limited utility in clinical practice. It is not an easy technique to perform, especially if the intubator has small hands. Nor is it aesthetically pleasing. However, it should be a technique in the armamentarium of the emergency physician.

B. Indications and contraindications

Digital intubation may be indicated:

- In situations with poor lighting, difficult patient position, disrupted airway anatomy, or potential C-spine instability. Many of these situations are more likely in prehospital situations (e.g., a patient trapped in an automobile)
- If equipment to do the laryngoscopy is unavailable or not working
- When visualization of the larynx is impossible (e.g. blood, secretions)
- In failed intubation

Patients must be sufficiently obtunded to prevent a biting injury to the intubator.

C. Technique

1. Have an assistant use a gauze sponge to gently but firmly retract the tongue.
2. Insert a stylet in the ETT and bend the ETT/stylet at a 90-degree angle at the junction of the middle and distal thirds of the tube.
3. Slide the index and long fingers of the nondominant hand palm down along the tongue.
4. Identify the tip of the epiglottis with the tip of the long finger and direct it anteriorly.
5. Insert the ETT/stylet in the mouth and use the index finger to direct it into the glottic opening.

D. Success rates and complications

Perhaps the most substantial limitation in performing this technique successfully is the length of the intubator's fingers relative to the patient's oropharyngeal dimensions.

Biting injuries or unintentional dental injuries to the hand with the risk of infectious disease transmission may occur.

The technique has only infrequently been used in the ED.

E. Tips and pearls

Remember to have an assistant retract the tongue to allow the intubator best access to the epiglottis. Sacchetti has recommended this technique for premature and newborn infants.

IV. Laryngeal mask airway

A. Definition

The laryngeal mask airway (LMA) was designed by the British anesthesiologist Archie Brain and has been referred to as the "Brain airway." The LMA looks like an ETT with an inflatable, elliptical, silicone rubber collar ("laryngeal mask") at the bottom end. The device is designed to surround and cover the supraglottic area, providing upper-airway continuity. Two rubber bars cross the tube opening at the mask end to prevent herniation of the epiglottis into the tube.

The original LMA design (known as the classic LMA) is available in disposable and multiuse formats. A new device that facilitates blind endotracheal intubation is known as the Fastrach LMA or the intubating laryngeal mask (ILM). The ILM has incorporated an epiglottic elevating bar and a ramp that directs an ETT up and into the larynx, enhancing the success rate of blind intubation. The ILM device is a substantial advance in airway management, particularly as a rescue device in the "can't intubate, can't oxygenate" situation while preparations for cricothyrotomy are under way.

The devices are easy to use, produce little in the way of adverse cardiovascular responses on insertion, and are useful in a limited way in emergency airway management. However, they do not constitute *definitive airway management,* unless one is successful at passing an ETT through the device into the trachea. They do not prevent regurgitation of gastric contents, nor do they protect the airway from aspiration. The patient must be significantly obtunded to tolerate insertion of these devices. The original LMA device and the ILM or Fastrach are fairly expensive but can be autoclaved and reused. The disposable device is less expensive and nonreusable but is not available in the "intubating" configuration. For ED use, the ILM is the recommended device, along with its specially modified ETT, because it results in a high incidence of successful tracheal intubation.

B. Indications and contraindications

The LMA is now widely used in anesthetic practice instead of mask anesthesia. In emergency practice it is used as a temporizing measure in a failed-airway situation. Provided laryngeal pathology is not the reason for airway obstruction, the LMA or ILM is often capable of establishing an airway, permitting gas exchange while one plans definitive airway management.

The patient must be deeply sedated or unconscious to insert the device.

C. Technique: classic LMA

Select the appropriate size of LMA: #3 in teenagers and small adult females; #4 and #5 in average-sized and large adults. Smaller sizes are available for use in infants and children.

1. Lubricate both sides of the LMA with water-soluble lubricant to facilitate insertion. Completely deflate the cuff and ensure that it is not folded.
2. Open the airway by using a head tilt as one would in basic airway management, if possible.
3. Insert the LMA into the mouth with the laryngeal surface down. Press the device onto the hard palate and advance it over the back of the tongue, using the curve of the device to follow the natural curve of the oro- and hypopharynx, to facilitate its falling into position over the larynx. The dimensions and design of the device allow it to wedge into the esophagus with gentle caudad pressure and to stop in the appropriate position over the larynx.
4. Inflate the collar with air (20 ml #3; 30 ml #4; 40 ml #5), or until there is no leak with bag ventilation.

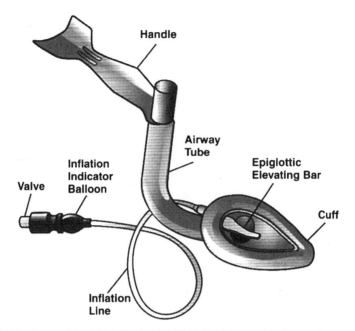

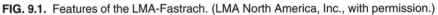

FIG. 9.1. Features of the LMA-Fastrach. (LMA North America, Inc., with permission.)

D. Technique: ILM (Fig. 9.1)

   1. Lubricate both sides of the ILM with water-soluble lubricant to facilitate insertion. Deflate cuff and ensure that it is not folded.

   2. Open the airway by using a head tilt as one would in basic airway management, if possible.

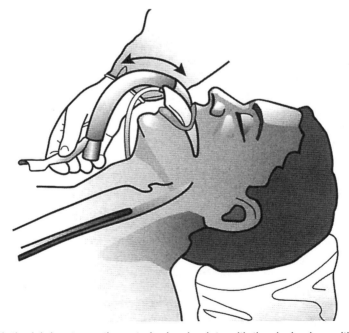

FIG. 9.2. Rub the lubricant over the anterior hard palate with the device in position as shown here. (LMA North America, Inc., with permission.)

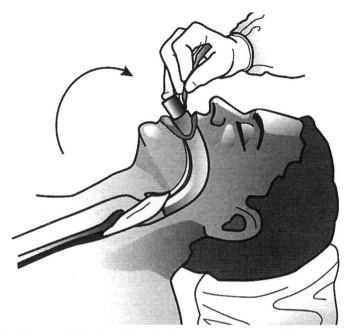

FIG. 9.3. Swing the mask into place in a circular movement, maintaining pressure against the palate and posterior pharynx. (LMA North America, Inc., with permission.)

    3. Grasp the metal handle of the ILM and insert the device straight back over the tongue to the back of the oropharynx. Then rotate the device using the metal handle over the back of the tongue into position. Once in place, inflate the collar to achieve a seal with bag-and-mask ventilation (Figs. 9.2 through 9.4). The metal handle may be used to manipulate the device to achieve a seal.

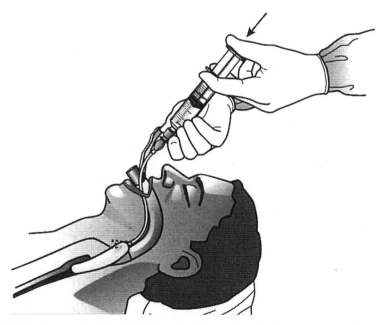

FIG. 9.4. Inflate the mask, without holding the tube or handle, to a pressure of approximately 60 cm H_2O (LMA North America, Inc., with permission.)

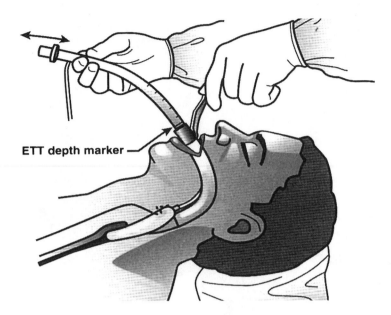

FIG. 9.5. Hold the LMA-Fastrach handle steady while gently inserting the ETT into the metal shaft up to the 15-cm transverse depth marker. (LMA North America, Inc., with permission.)

4. Once adequate oxygen saturations have been established, the silicone-tipped, armored ETT supplied with the ILM can be used to attempt intubation. Lubricate the tube well. With the black vertical line on the tube facing the operator, insert the ETT into the metal tube of the ILM until the horizontal black line on the ETT is at the

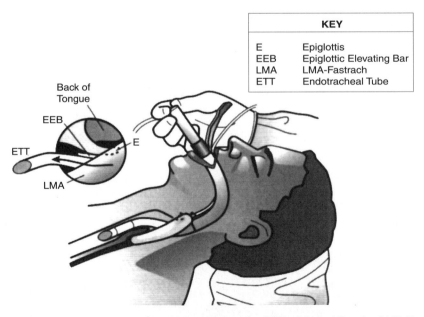

KEY	
E	Epiglottis
EEB	Epiglottic Elevating Bar
LMA	LMA-Fastrach
ETT	Endotracheal Tube

FIG. 9.6. If no resistance is felt, continue to advance the ETT while holding the LMA-Fastrach steady until intubation has been accomplished. Key: **E,** Epiglottis; **EEB,** Epiglottic Elevating Bar; **LMA,** LMA-Fastrach; **ETT,** Endotracheal Tube. (LMA North America, Inc., with permission.)

proximal entrance to the ILM. At this point, the tip of the ETT is at the glottic opening of the ILM (Fig. 9.5). Resistance will be felt as the ETT is advanced through the end of the ILM and into the glottis (Fig. 9.6). Verification of endotracheal placement may be accomplished by using a lightwand, carbon dioxide detection, or other means. First-pass success rates of 70% to 80% are reported. Manipulation of the ILM by the metal handle may enhance successful passage in the event of failure. The most useful maneuver appears to be a short (1- to 2-cm) withdrawal then reinsertion of the ILM.

5. The ILM can be deflated and left in situ, or withdrawn over the ETT. A stabilizing wand is provided with the ILM ETT to hold the ETT in position while the ILM is withdrawn, preventing the displacement of the ETT (Figs. 9.7 through 9.11).

E. **Success rates and complications**

The LMA does not prevent the aspiration of gastric contents, serving to emphasize its role as a temporizing measure only. This limits its usefulness in prehospital and emergency airway care, except when the ILM is used to facilitate endotracheal intubation.

There is no literature describing the success rate of this device in the ED.

F. **Tips and pearls**

- Partial inflation of the cuff to make it slightly firm may facilitate insertion. Some reports have advocated insertion with the cuff fully inflated.
- Use of a laryngoscope may facilitate insertion.
- Some individuals prefer to insert the device upside down, like an oropharyngeal airway, and then to rotate the device 180 degrees in the posterior oropharynx into position. This technique does not appear advantageous.
- A lightwand with the rigid, internal stylette removed, may be passed through the ILM to demonstrate tracheal entrance; then the ETT may be passed over the lightwand.

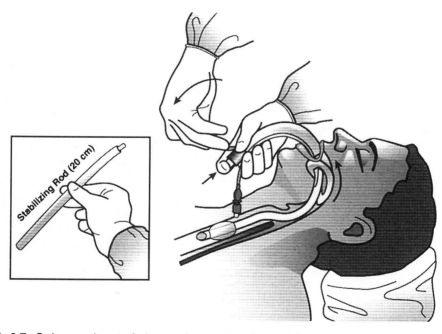

FIG. 9.7. Swing mask out of pharynx into oral cavity, applying counterpressure to tracheal tube with finger as shown prior to insertion of a stabilizing rod. (LMA North America, Inc., with permission.)

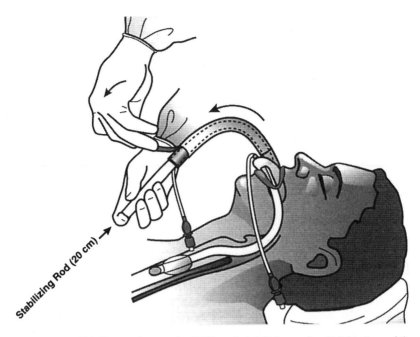

FIG. 9.8. Slide the LMA-Fastrach over the ETT and stabilizing rod until it is clear of the mouth. (LMA North America, Inc., with permission.)

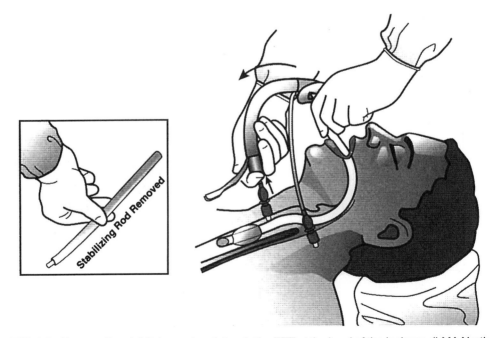

FIG. 9.9. Remove the stabilizing rod and steady the ETT at the level of the incisors. (LMA North America, Inc., with permission.)

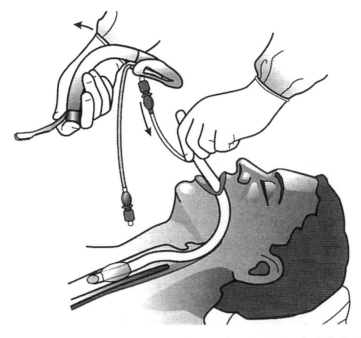

FIG. 9.10. Remove the LMA-Fastrach completely, gently unthreading the inflation line and pilot balloon of the ETT. (LMA North America, Inc., with permission.)

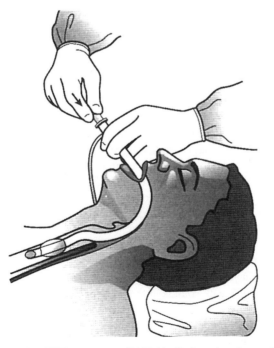

FIG. 9.11. Replace the ETT connector. (LMA North America, Inc., with permission.)

V. The esophageal/tracheal Combitube
A. Definition
The Combitube is a dual-lumen, dual-cuff airway invented by Michael Frass, an Austrian intensivist. The Combitube, in the context of ED airway management, is a rescue airway device. It has two lumens, allowing ventilation whether placed into the esophagus or the trachea. It is a dramatic improvement over the esophageal obturator airway, which has no place in modern emergency airway management. In addition, unlike its predecessors the esophageal obturator airway (EOA) and the esophageal gastric tube airway (EGTA), an adequate mask seal is unnecessary to effect adequate ventilation. A large, eccentric oropharyngeal balloon provides a sufficient seal to permit ventilation through distal apertures.

The Combitube is supplied in two sizes: 37F SA (small adult), to be used in patients 4 to 6 feet tall, and 41 F, which is for use in patients more than 6 feet tall. Combitubes suitable for use in pediatrics are unavailable.

B. Indications and contraindications
1. Indications
   - Failed intubation, particularly the "can't intubate, can't ventilate" situation in which the etiology is felt *not* to be due to upper-airway obstruction at the level of the larynx and cricothyrotomy is not immediately possible.
   - Primary airway management for cardiopulmonary arrest when ET intubation is not permitted or impossible (e.g., prehospital care).
2. Contraindications
   - Responsive patients with intact airway-protective reflexes
   - Patients with known esophageal disease
   - Caustic ingestions
   - Upper-airway obstruction due to laryngeal foreign bodies or pathology

C. Technique
Insertion of the Combitube is a blind technique, though a laryngoscope may be used, permitting insertion under direct vision:
1. With the patient in the supine position (insertion is possible in any position), lift the tongue and jaw upward with the nondominant hand.
2. Insert the device in the midline, allowing the curve of the device to follow the natural curve of the airway and advance the device until the alveolar ridge is opposite imprinted bands on the device. Force is not necessary to seat the device correctly. Resistance should prompt the operator to withdraw and readvance.
3. Inflate the proximal, large oropharyngeal balloon with approximately 100 ml of air (Combitube 37F: 85 ml) via the blue pilot balloon labeled #1.
4. Inflate the white, distal balloon with 5 to 15 ml of air (Combitube 37F: 5 to 12 ml) via the white pilot balloon labeled #2.
5. Begin ventilation using the longer, blue connecting tube.
6. The presence of air entry into the lung and the absence of gastric insufflation by auscultation indicates that the Combitube is in the esophagus, which occurs virtually all the time. Aspiration of gastric contents, and gastric decompression, is possible by passing a tube through the clear connecting tube into the stomach.
7. The absence of breath sounds in the chest and presence of gastric insufflation by auscultation indicates that the Combitube is in the trachea (a distinctly rare event) and ventilation should be performed through the shorter, clear connection tube.
8. The absence of any sounds on auscultation may indicate that the device has been inserted too far and should be repositioned after the proximal balloon is deflated.

9. End-tidal carbon dioxide verification should be used to ensure pulmonary gas exchange.

D. Success rates and complications

The Combitube has been shown to be an effective airway management device. It is not difficult to position properly. The Combitube appears in one study to be superior to the EGTA and the LMA in the prehospital setting, and it has been shown to be a useful airway rescue device in the event of a failed intubation. However, like the LMA, it does not provide optimum protection against aspiration (although aspiration has never been reported), and its merit relative to the ILM is unknown. A high rate of success with few complications have been reported in prehospital use for cardiac arrest.

E. Tips and pearls

Do not apply excessive force to the tube during insertion. Perforation of the vallecula, pyriform recess, and esophagus has been reported.

Insert the provided suction catheter into the stomach as soon as the device is placed to reduce the risk of pulmonary aspiration.

ADDITIONAL READING

Blostein PA, Koestner AJ, Hoak S. Failed rapid sequence intubation in trauma patients: oesophageal tracheal Combitube is a useful adjunct. *J Trauma* 1998;44:534–537.

DeMello WF, Kocan M. The laryngeal mask in failed intubation. *Anaesthesia* 1990;45:689.

Dhara SS. Retrograde intubation: a facilitated approach. *Br J Anaesth* 1992;69:631.

Frass M. The Combitube: oesophageal/tracheal double lumen airway. In: Benumof JL, ed. *Airway management: principles and practice.* St Louis: Mosby, 1996.

Hardwick WC, Bluhm D. Digital intubation. *J Emerg Med* 1984;1:317.

Hung OR, Murphy MF. Lightwands, lighted stylets and blind techniques of intubation. In: Sandler AN, Doyle DJ, eds. The difficult airway. *Anaesthesia Clinics NA,* vol 13, Toronto: WB Saunders, 1995.

Hung OR, Pytka S, Murphy MF, et al. Comparative hemodynamic changes following laryngoscopic or lightwand intubation. *Anesthesiology* 1993;79:A497.

Hung OR, Stevens SC, Pytka S, et al. Clinical trial of a new lightwand device for intubation in patients with difficult airways. *Anesthesiology* 1993;79:A498.

Joshi GP, Smith I, White PF. Laryngeal mask airway. In: Benumof JL, ed. *Airway management: principles and practice.* St Louis: Mosby, 1996.

Korber TE, Henneman PC. Digital nasotracheal intubation. *J Emerg Med* 1989;7:275.

Murphy, MF. Blind digital intubation. In: Benumof JL, ed. *Airway management: principles and practice.* St Louis: Mosby, 1996.

Shantha TR. Retrograde intubation using the subcricoid region. *BJA* 1992;68:109.

Stewart RD. Tactile orotracheal intubation. *Ann Emerg Med* 1984;13:175.

Tanagawa K, Shigematsu A. Choice of airway devices for 12,020 cases of nontraumatic cardiac arrest in Japan. *Prehosp Emerg Care* 1998;2:96–100.

Wissler RN. The oesophageal-tracheal Combitube. *Anaesth Rev* 1993;20:147.

Woody NC, Woody HB. Direct digital intubation for neonatal resuscitation. *J Pediatr* 1968;73:903.

10

Fiberoptic Intubation Techniques

Michael F. Murphy

*Departments of Emergency Medicine and Anaesthesiology, Queen Elizabeth II
Health Sciences Centre, Dalhousie University, Halifax, Nova Scotia*

Although a discussion of difficult airway management is not complete without a review of the use of fiberoptic equipment to effect intubation, few emergency physicians and emergency departments (EDs) are equipped for this procedure. In addition, there is little literature on fiberoptic-assisted intubation in the ED. However, the skill is an important one for the emergency physician, both to facilitate endotracheal intubation of the difficult airway and to perform diagnostic and therapeutic procedures on the upper airway. Fiberoptic intubation underwent a similar development in anesthesia, and increasing ED use can be anticipated.

I. Intubating fiberoptic scopes
A. Definition

Endotracheal intubation over a fiberoptic bronchoscope has emerged as an invaluable technique in airway management, particularly in patients in which standard laryngoscopy and orotracheal intubation have failed or are anticipated to be difficult or impossible. Fiberoptic intubation requires considerable technical skill that needs continual exposure to maintain speed and success. In addition, maximal success rates with this technique require both psychologic and pharmacologic patient preparation. When the procedure is to be done awake, the patient who knows what to expect, is sedated, and has had an antisialogogue administered has the optimum chance for success. The emergency situation is usually much different.

Instrument selection for the ED is an important issue. Affordable and durable scopes are now available. These instruments, although expensive, find several uses in the ED:

- Endotracheal intubation
- Diagnostic laryngoscopy
- Oropharyngeal foreign-body location and extraction
- Pulmonary toilette

The scope should be of sufficient caliber and stiffness to allow intubation over itself without kinking, while at the same time maintaining flexibility and ease of manipulation. The scope should be small enough to allow passage through a topically anesthetized nose for diagnostic work. A 4- to 4.5-mm outside-diameter (OD) fiberoptic scope is best. Some manufacturers reinforce the smaller scopes to enhance their rigidity, facilitating passage of an endotracheal tube (ETT) into the glottis over the scope.

The scope should be of sufficient length (60 cm) to allow bronchoscopy and airway toilette in the ED. A separate channel for the insufflation of oxygen, the injection of local anesthetic or saline, and suctioning is essential. A new generation of fiberoptic scopes with battery-powered self-contained light sources promises to be much more compact and may be preferable for ED applications.

B. Indications and contraindications

   1. Indications:
   - Predicted difficult intubation
   - C-spine immobility required
   - Anatomic abnormalities
   - Failed intubation in the "can't intubate, can oxygenate" scenario

   2. Contraindications:
   - Excessive blood and secretions in the upper airway have the great potential to obscure the view and reduce the success rate with the fiberoptic technique (relative)
   - Upper-airway obstruction due to foreign bodies or other lesions (relative)
   - Inadequate oxygenation by bag and mask does not permit fiberoptic intubation because of the time required (absolute)

C. Care and use of the instrument

Some general precautions to prevent damage to the scope and its relatively delicate fiberoptic bundles:

   1. Don't drop the scope.
   2. Use a bite-block (e.g., oral airway) to protect the scope. A convenient "break-away" bite block is available.
   3. Avoid acute bending or kinking, especially when sliding the ETT over the scope into the trachea.
   4. If rotation of the ETT during intubation is necessary, rotate both the ETT and the scope to avoid damage to the fibers.
   5. Lubricate the ETT by spraying local anesthetic agent or other water-soluble material down the tube to allow easy removal of the scope after the ETT is in place. Lubricating the scope makes it slippery and difficult to manipulate.
   6. Clean the working channel immediately after use.
   7. Don't flex the tip against undue resistance or use it to move tissue out of the way.

D. Technique

The operator should be familiar with the equipment and have had the opportunity to practice on mannequins before managing an emergency case. The manufacturers of fiberscopes have training videos, sales personnel, and mannequins that provide a good introduction to the technique. Recent studies have shown that the technique can also be learned in real-life situations by the performance of upper-airway endoscopy when diagnostic opportunities, such as foreign bodies, hoarseness, and other upper-airway conditions present themselves. Semiemergent intubations, such as overdose victims that are easily ventilated and have a normal oxygen saturation, may be appropriate candidates for fiberoptic intubation.

Scope tip control is simple: Flexion forward and backward is achieved with the thumb lever on the handle; rotation clockwise and counterclockwise is done by rotating the wrist (not the entire upper body).

Preparation for the task depends on how much time is available. Generally, most things should be in a state of instantaneous readiness:

   1. Gather all your equipment (usually preassembled on a tray):
   - Topical airway anesthesia supplies and equipment
   - Scope, ETTs, airways, bite-blocks
   - Tonsil suction

- Lubricant and silicone liquid drops (prevents fogging)
- Additional airway management equipment as indicated in case of patient deterioration and need for rapid intervention

2. Obtain an able assistant.
3. Prepare the patient:
   - Antisialogogue, such as glycopyrrolate 0.01 mg/kg intramuscularly (IM) (or intravenously [IV])
   - "Judicious sedation" if appropriate
   - Topical anesthesia
   - Vasoconstrictor for the nose (if nasal route chosen)
   - Administer supplemental oxygen if needed
4. Lubricate the tube (as earlier) and slide it over the scope up to the handpiece. Jam the ETT connector to the handpiece to hold it in place. Lubricating the scope makes it slippery and too hard to manipulate.
5. Put a drop of silicone liquid on the tip of the scope to prevent fogging.
6. Put in bite-block (if oral route is chosen).
7. Stand up straight at the head of the bed. Move your hands and arms, not your torso.
8. Stay in the midline, stay in the midline, stay in the midline! Custom-made airways such as Ovassapian and Berman Breakaway Airways are very helpful in accomplishing this. If these adjuncts are used, insert the ETT through the airway and then insert the scope through the airway/ETT combination, obviating the need to jam the ETT connector onto the scope handpiece.
9. Hold the body of the fiberscope in your dominant hand using your thumb to toggle the tip control lever up and down. Your nondominant hand advances, withdraws, and manipulates the scope. Maintain gentle tension between your hands to permit left and right rotation of the tip.
10. Nasal technique: Advance the nasal tube to the nasopharynx and then pass the scope through the tube.
11. Oral technique: Use the little finger of your free "scope hand" to feel the lower lip and keep you in the midline. Gentle traction on the tongue by an assistant helps open the airway and prevent the patient from using the tongue to obstruct access to the airway. This assistant should have a tonsil suction available to aspirate oral secretions. The working channel of the scope may provide insufficient suction to clear the volume of secretions that are usually present during the procedure.
12. Get your bearings: The base of the tongue is "up"; advance slowly while flexing the tip up to pass over the back of the tongue. The epiglottis comes into view. Keep it "above" you. You will see the white cords opening and closing with respiration.
13. It is hard to time it, but try to advance the scope through the cords during inspiration. You may need to inject 2 to 4 ml of 4% lidocaine through the working channel onto the larynx to obtund the cough or closure reflex. Have 4 ml of 4% lidocaine drawn up and ready in case you need it to get through the cords.
14. If you get lost, withdraw to the oropharynx and find a landmark.
15. If secretions or blood are plentiful and not cleared by suctioning through the working channel, have your assistant suction with a tonsil suction through the mouth.
16. Once you are through the cords advance the scope down into the trachea, being careful not to hit the carina and stimulate coughing. Now slowly advance the ETT and the scope together into the trachea. Be careful not to kink the scope. Gentle rotation of the scope/tube unit through 180 degrees may be necessary if it catches on the cords.

17. If coughing is a persistent problem, inject 2 to 3 ml of lidocaine 4% through the scope.

E. Instrument cleaning

Department policies related to cleaning and storage of the scope must be developed. Universal precautions are to be used in cleaning the instrument. Although the technique can be adapted easily from the endoscopy clinic or the operating room, the following is a sample routine:

1. Wipe outside surfaces with saline and a clean cloth to remove debris immediately after use.
2. Flush the working channel with 100 to 200 ml of saline immediately after use.
3. Soak for 15 minutes in a CIDEX bath, aspirating and injecting the working channel.
4. Rinse the scope and its channel thoroughly in sterile water.
5. Wipe the scope dry and store it.

F. Success rates and complications

Success depends on familiarity and skill in using the device and on patient selection and setting. The single study looking at fiberoptic intubation in the ED identified a 70% success rate after gaining some experience. In the hands of trained endoscopists, the success rate approaches 100%.

Patient complications with this technique are uncommon and include mucosal damage to the airway and epistaxis. As with all techniques, damage to the vocal apparatus is possible but rare. The most frequent complication is damage to the scope from biting, twisting, kinking, or dropping.

G. Tips and pearls

- Stand erect and keep some tension on the scope between the hands. This eliminates redundancy or slackness in the scope and permits clockwise and counterclockwise twisting of the wrist and body of the scope to be translated into similar motion at the tip of the scope.
- New users may not want to manipulate the scope/thumb toggle until the tip of the scope has been advanced into the hypopharynx. At this point, rotation and the toggle are used to keep the now visualized glottis in the center of the operator's view, "much like a video game."
- After intubation, the scope can be passed just distal to the end of the ETT, then flexed fully forward. Gradually, the tube/scope combination are withdrawn until the light of the scope transilluminates the trachea at the sternal notch. This confirms that the tube is in the midtrachea (where it should be) and the scope is then withdrawn while the tube is stabilized.
- Remember to use the little finger of the lower hand to keep you in the midline.
- Don't use too much lubricant.
- Some authorities advise the insufflation of oxygen through the working channel to maintain oxygenation and blow secretions out of the way during fiberoptic intubation. However, insufflation of the stomach to the point of rupture has been reported, so this is no longer recommended.

II. Bullard laryngoscope

A. Definition

The Bullard Laryngoscope (Circon ACMI Corp, Stamford, CT) is a fiberoptic device coupled with a nonmalleable intubating blade designed to fall into the appropriate intubating position on insertion into the hypopharynx. Thus it is basically a rigid fiberoptic laryngoscope. It was invented by the American anesthesiologist Roger Bullard. An ETT is mounted on a stylet that is also part of the device. Once placed, the device allows the intubator a direct, fiberoptically delivered view of the larynx. It is then possible to slide the stylet-mounted ETT into the airway under direct vision.

The fiberoptic nature and design of the device may be advantageous in those situations where mouth opening is limited or cervical spine motion is to be avoided. The operator sees the glottis via the fiberoptic eyepiece, and alignment of all the axes of intubation for direct visualization of the glottis is not required.

B. Indications and contraindications

1. Indications:
   - Predicted difficult intubation
   - C-spine immobility required
   - Failed intubation in the "can't intubate, can oxygenate" scenario
2. Contraindications:
   - Excessive blood and secretions in the upper airway can obscure the view and reduce the success rate with any fiberoptic technique; the Bullard laryngoscope is no exception
   - The design of the device is dependent on normal upper-airway anatomy to maximize success. Upper-airway obstruction due to foreign bodies or other lesions is a relative contraindication

C. Technique

- Attach the "blade extender" to the device
- Load the ETT onto the stylet with the stylet protruding through the Murphy eye. Some do not use the Murphy eye. It is worth noting that this is the only technique where a stylet is permitted to protrude beyond the end of the ETT due to the direct vision nature of the technique
- Lubricate the blade and tube
- Hold the device in the left hand
- The blade/stylet/ETT device is inserted into the mouth in the horizontal plane, over the top of the tongue, and then rotated caudad in the sagittal plane into the posterior pharynx. The device follows the natural curve of the oro- and hypopharynx, and force is unnecessary to place the device
- Visualize the epiglottis through the fiberoptic viewer as the device is advanced, pick it up, and lift it anteriorly. This is done by lifting the handle away from the chin and not by "fulcruming"
- Visualize the glottic opening and advance the ETT off the stylet into the airway

D. Success rates and complications

This device requires some practice, though those with experience with fiberoptic intubation catch onto the view presented and become orientated to the device relatively quickly. One center now has experience with more than 40 emergency intubations with the Bullard laryngoscope, and a multicenter trial is planned as part of the National Emergency Airway Registry.

Damage to teeth and airway structures is possible:

- If the device is forcefully inserted or manipulated
- If the tip of the stylet is not kept in view and prevented from skewering soft tissues

E. Tips and pearls

- Fully load the ETT onto the stylet to minimize the bulk of the device and the extent of mouth opening
- For adults use the "blade extender" that comes with the device to ensure that there is sufficient length to pick up the epiglottis

- Use a catheter on the mouth or nasal prongs to deliver oxygen in the spontaneously breathing patient and monitor SpO_2

III. Visualized EndoTracheal Tube (VETT)

A. Definition

The Visualized EndoTracheal Tube, or VETT (Pulmonx), is an ETT with a fiberoptic bundle and three light channels embedded in the tube. This device has only recently been approved by the Food and Drug Administration and experience is limited.

The embedded fiberoptic bundle can be attached to a uniquely designed video monitor or to special video goggles, allowing the operator to see what the end of the ETT sees. With the appropriate shaping of the tube and the proper insertion technique, the tube can be maneuvered into the larynx and trachea under direct vision.

B. Indications and contraindications

1. Indications:
   - Predicted difficult intubation
   - C-spine immobility required
   - Failed intubation in the "can't intubate, can oxygenate" scenario
2. Contraindications:
   - Excessive blood and secretions in the upper airway may obscure the view and reduce the success rate with any fiberoptic technique; the VETT is no exception

C. Technique

Although the device allows direct vision intubation, the technique of intubation is more similar to that described for the lightwand than any of the fiberoptic techniques described earlier:

1. *Preparation.* The ETT embedded with the fiberoptic bundle should be bent just proximal to the endotracheal cuff, into a right angle, mimicking the shape of a "field hockey stick" with the aid of a stylet. The tip of the ETT should also be lubricated with a water-soluble lubricant.

2. *Positioning.* With the intubator standing at the head of the patient, the neck is bared to allow maximal visualization of the anterior neck of the patient during intubation. Like the lightwand, transillumination in the midline anteriorly at the level of the cricothyroid membrane is a useful adjunctive observation in placing the VETT in the trachea. The technique can also be performed from the side of the patient. Usually, the patient's head and neck are placed in a neutral position, though it may be necessary to extend the head slightly to optimize visualization. In obese patients or patients with an extremely short neck, placing a pillow under the shoulder and neck may be helpful.

3. *Technique of intubation.* With the patient lying supine, the lower alveolar ridge and mentum are grasped and lifted upward using the intubator's nondominant hand. This lifts the tongue and epiglottis upward to facilitate the intubation. The nondominant hand must be kept close to the lower lip to ensure an unobstructed path in the midline for the lightwand. The device is inserted into the oropharynx and positioned in the midline. The device is then rocked back and forth in the midline in an imaginary arc that is anticipated to allow successful placement of the VETT in the glottis, while observing at the same time the view on the monitor or goggles and using this view as an aid to directing the rocking motion. The jaw lift helps to elevate the epiglottis and enhance the passage of the VETT under the epiglottis into the airway. When the tip of the VETT enters the glottic opening, a well-defined circumscribed glow can be seen at the anterior neck slightly below the laryngeal prominence. The rigid stylet is removed and the tip of the ETT is

advanced until the glow from the fiberoptic bundle appears in the sternal notch. At this point, the tip of the ETT is midway between the vocal cords and carina.

D. Success rates and complications

Studies using the VETT have demonstrated high success rates in the hands of skilled airway managers. There is little literature to date on its use in the emergency department setting. However, the innovative design presents a compelling case for a role for this device in emergency airway management in the future.

E. Tips and pearls

- Maintain gentle upward traction on the mandible
- Place the monitor in an easily seen location or wear the goggles
- Combine the advantage of direct vision with the technique of transillumination
- Rock the VETT gently back and forth in the midline; force is not necessary
- Place the bend in the VETT just proximal to the balloon of the ETT in normal individuals, more proximally in those with long necks, more distally in those with short necks. Make a good right-angle bend

ADDITIONAL READING

Afilalo M, Guttman A, Stern E, et al. Fiberoptic intubation in the emergency department: a case series. *J Emerg Med* 1993;11:387–391.

Cooper SD, Benumoff JL, Ozaki QT, et al. Evaluation of the Bullard laryngoscope using the new intubating stylet: comparison with conventional laryngoscopy. *Anesth Analg* 1994;79:965.

Delaney KA, Hessler R. Emergency flexible fiberoptic nasotracheal intubation. A report of 60 cases. *Ann Emerg Med* 1988;17:919–926.

Messeter MD, Pettersson KI. Endotracheal intubation with the fiberoptic bronchoscope. *Anaesthesia* 1980;35: 294–298.

Mlinek EJ, Clinton JE, Plummer D, et al. Fiberoptic intubation in the emergency department. *Ann Emerg Med* 1990; 19:359–362.

Mulder DS, Wallace DH, Woolhouse FM. The use of the fiberoptic bronchoscope to facilitate endotracheal intubation following head and neck trauma. *J Trauma* 1975;15:638–640.

Schafermeyer RW. Fiberoptic laryngoscopy in the emergency department. *Am J Emerg Med* 1984;2:160–163.

Shigemastsu T, Miyazawa N, Kobayashi M, et al. Nasal intubation with the Bullard laryngoscope: a useful approach for difficult airways. *Anesth Analg* 1994;79:132.

11

Surgical Airway Techniques

Ron M. Walls* and Robert J. Vissers†

*Chairman, Department of Emergency Medicine, Brigham and Women's Hospital,
Associate Professor of Medicine, Division of Emergency Medicine,
Harvard Medical School, Boston, Massachusetts; †Department of Emergency Medicine,
University of North Carolina, Chapel Hill, North Carolina

I. Surgical airway management

Surgical airway management is defined as the creation of an airway by surgical techniques. All other methods of airway management utilize existing portals of access to the trachea. Surgical airway management involves the creation of an opening to the trachea by surgical means and the use of this opening to provide ventilation and oxygenation. There is some confusion engendered by use of the term *surgical airway management*. In some discussions, surgical airway management includes both cricothyrotomy and needle cricothyrotomy with percutaneous transtracheal ventilation. Other discussions limit *surgical airway* to cricothyrotomy and consider percutaneous transtracheal ventilation to be simply another airway management technique. For the purposes of discussion in this chapter, *surgical airway management* is deemed to include cricothyrotomy, percutaneous transtracheal ventilation, and placement of a surgical airway using a cricothyrotome, which is a device intended to place a surgical airway percutaneously without performance of formal cricothyrotomy. The cricothyrotomes may be considered as an alternative to cricothyrotomy, but none of the available cricothyrotomes places a cuffed endotracheal tube (ETT) in the trachea, and so they do not afford airway protection. Similarly, percutaneous transtracheal ventilation does not protect the airway and should be considered a temporizing measure only. In children 12 years of age or under, however, percutaneous transtracheal ventilation is the method of choice for surgical airway management because of the technical difficulties of cricothyrotomy and cricothyrotome placement (see later). Each of the surgical airway techniques is described in detail in the sections that follow.

A. Definitions

Cricothyrotomy is the establishment of a surgical opening in the airway through the cricothyroid membrane and placement of a cuffed tracheostomy tube or ETT.

A cricothyrotome is a kit or device that is intended to establish a surgical airway without resorting to formal cricothyrotomy. These kits use two basic approaches. One approach is the Seldinger technique, in which the airway is accessed via a small needle through which a flexible guidewire is passed. The airway device is then passed over this guidewire and into the airway in a manner analogous with that of central line placement by the Seldinger technique. The other technique is the direct placement of an airway via a percutaneous device without the Seldinger technique. There have been no clinical studies to date demonstrating the superiority of any one approach over another or of any of these devices over formal surgical cricothyrotomy.

B. Indications and contraindications

The primary indication for cricothyrotomy is failure of intubation by oral or nasal means in the presence of an immediate need for definitive airway management. A second indication is a method of primary airway management in patients for whom nasotracheal or orotracheal intubation is contraindicated or felt to be impossible. Thus cricothyrotomy should be thought of as a rescue technique in most circumstances and only infrequently will be used as the primary method of airway management. An example of a circumstance in which cricothyrotomy would be the primary method of airway management is the patient with severe lower facial trauma in whom access through the mouth or nose will be difficult or impossible. This patient requires immediate airway management because of the risk of aspiration of blood and secretions, and cricothyrotomy is indicated. The algorithmic guidelines in Chapter 3 demonstrate the role of surgical airway management in the context of failed intubation or failed ventilation. Contraindications for surgical airway management are few and, with one exception, are relative. That one exception is young age. Children have a small, pliable, mobile larynx and cricoid cartilage, making cricothyrotomy extremely difficult. For children under 12 years of age, unless they are teenage or adult sized, percutaneous transtracheal ventilation should be used as the surgical airway management technique of choice. Other contraindications include preexisting laryngeal or tracheal pathology such as tumor, infections, or abscess in the area in which the procedure will be performed; hematoma or other anatomic destruction of the landmarks that would render the procedure difficult or impossible; coagulopathy; and lack of operator expertise. Cricothyrotomy has been performed successfully after systemic thrombolytic therapy for acute MI. Cricothyrotomy has a very high success rate when performed in the emergency department (ED) setting. The presence of an anatomic barrier in particular should prompt consideration of alternative techniques that might result in a successful airway. However, in cases in which no alternative method of airway management is likely to be successful or timely enough, cricothyrotomy should be performed without hesitation. The same principles apply for both the cricothyrotome and for percutaneous transtracheal ventilation. Percutaneous transtracheal ventilation is not contraindicated in small children and, in fact, is the surgical airway method of choice for children under 12 years of age. The cricothyrotomes have not been demonstrated to improve success rates or time, or to decrease complication rates when compared with surgical cricothyrotomy. As with formal cricothyrotomy, experience, skill, knowledge of anatomy, and adherence to proper technique are essential for success when a cricothyrotome is used.

II. Cricothyrotomy

A. Description and technique

The anterior neck should be prepared as much as is possible and care taken to identify the cricothyroid membrane correctly. The cricothyrotomy instrument set should be simple, consisting of only that equipment necessary to complete the procedure. A sample listing of recommended contents of a cricothyrotomy tray is shown in Box 11.1.

1. Identify the landmarks

The cricothyroid membrane is best identified by palpating the laryngeal prominence, which is the palpable protuberance at the anterior superior aspect of the larynx. The thyrohyoid space, which lies above the laryngeal prominence, and the hyoid bone, which resides high in the neck, should also be identified. This will prevent inadvertent identification of the thyrohyoid membrane as the cricothyroid membrane, which would lead to misplacement of the tracheostomy tube above the

---

Box 11.1.   Recommended contents of cricothyrotomy tray

a. Trousseau dilator
b. Tracheal hook
c. Scalpel with #11 blade
d. Cuffed, nonfenestrated, #4 Shiley tracheostomy tube
e. Optional equipment may include several 4 × 4 gauze sponges, two small hemostats, and surgical drapes.

---

vocal cords. Approximately one of the patient's finger breadths inferior to the laryngeal prominence is a small depression bounded on its inferior aspect by a rigid, horizontal structure. This small depression is the cricothyroid membrane and the rigid structure below it is the cricoid cartilage (Fig. 11.1). In difficult circumstances, the location of the cricothyroid membrane can be approximated by placing the four fingers of the operator's right hand together with the tip of the small finger in the sternal notch and the tips of the four fingers oriented vertically up the anterior midline of the neck. With the hand thus placed, the index finger will lie approximately over the cricothyroid membrane and this landmark should be used as the center point of the vertical anterior skin incision.

2. Prepare the neck

If time permits, apply appropriate antiseptic solution. Local anesthesia is desirable if the patient is conscious. Infiltration of the skin and subcutaneous tissue of the anterior neck with 1% lidocaine solution will provide adequate anesthesia.

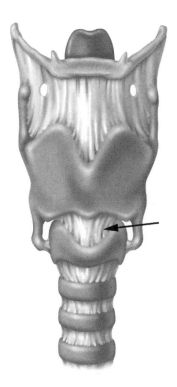

FIG. 11.1. Anatomy of the larynx. The cricothyroid membrane (*arrow*) is bordered above by the thyroid cartilage and below by the cricoid cartilage.

3. Immobilize the larynx

Throughout the procedure, the larynx must be immobilized (Fig. 11.2). This is best done by placing the thumb and long finger on opposite sides of the superior laryngeal horns, the posterior superior aspect of the laryngeal cartilage. With the thumb and long finger thus placed, the index finger is ideally positioned anteriorly to relocate and reidentify the cricothyroid membrane at any time during the procedure.

4. Incise the skin

A generously sized vertical midline incision should be used (Fig. 11.3). This incision should be approximately 2 cm in length and should extend down to but not through any of the deep structures of the neck. The cricothyroid membrane is separated from the outside world only by skin, subcutaneous tissue, and anterior cervical fascia. Care must be taken with the incision to incise this tissue only and not to extend the incision into the larynx, through the cricothyroid membrane, or through the cricoid cartilage or the trachea.

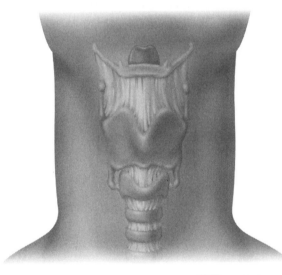

A

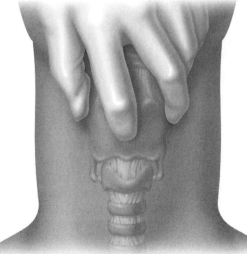

FIG. 11.2. A: Surface anatomy of the airway. **B:** The thumb and long finger immobilize the superior cornua of the larynx; the index finger palpates the cricothyroid membrane.

B

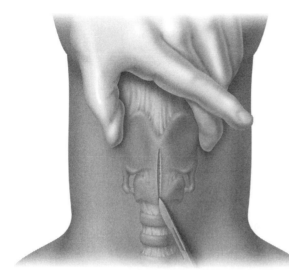

FIG. 11.3. With the index finger moved to the side but continued firm immobilization of the larynx, a vertical, midline skin incision is made, down to the depth of the laryngeal structures.

5. Reidentify the membrane

With the thumb and long finger maintaining immobilization of the larynx, the index finger can now palpate the anterior larynx, the cricothyroid membrane, and the cricoid cartilage without any interposed skin or subcutaneous tissue (Fig. 11.4). The landmarks thus confirmed, the index finger can be left in the wound by placing it on the inferior aspect of the anterior larynx, thus providing a clear indicator of the superior extent of the cricothyroid membrane.

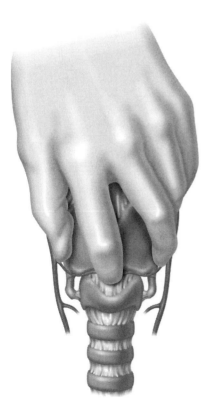

FIG. 11.4. With skin incised, the index finger can now directly palpate the cricothyroid membrane.

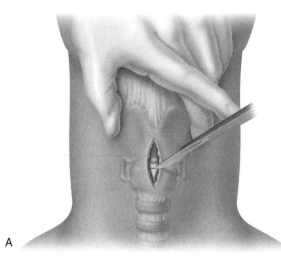

A

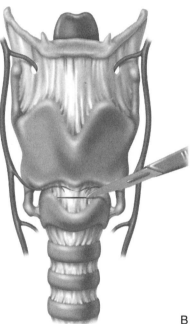

FIG. 11.5. A: A horizontal membrane incision is made near the inferior edge of the cricothyroid membrane. The index finger may be swung aside or may remain in the wound, palpating the inferior edge of the thyroid cartilage, to "guide" the scalpel to the membrane. **B:** A low cricothyroid incision avoids the superior cricothyroid vessels, which run transversely near the top of the membrane.

B

6. Incise the membrane

   The cricothyroid membrane should be incised in a horizontal direction, with an incision at least 1 cm long (Fig. 11.5A). It is recommended to try to incise the lower half of the membrane rather than the upper half because of the relatively superior location of the superior cricothyroid artery and vein (Fig. 11.5B).

7. Insert the tracheal hook

   The tracheal hook is then turned so that it is oriented in the transverse plane, passed through the incision, and turned so that the hook is oriented in a cephalad direction. The hook is then applied to the inferior aspect of the thyroid cartilage, and light upward and anterior traction is applied to bring the airway immediately out to the skin incision (Fig. 11.6). If an assistant is available, this hook may be passed to the assistant to maintain immobilization of the larynx.

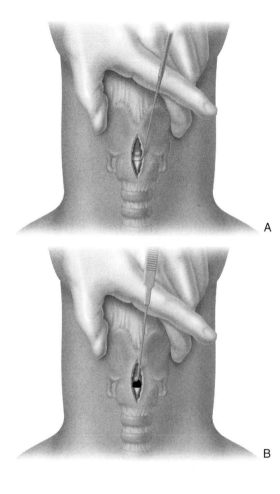

A

B

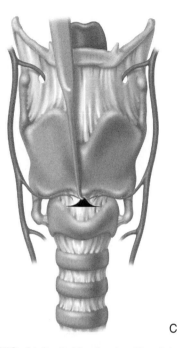

C

FIG. 11.6. A: The tracheal hook is oriented transversely during insertion. **B, C:** After insertion, cephalad traction is applied to the inferior margin of the thyroid cartilage.

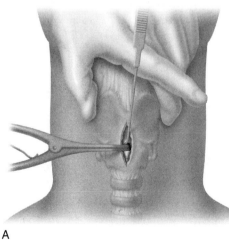

A

FIG. 11.7. A: Trousseau dilator inserted a short distance into the incision. **B:** In this orientation, the dilator enlarges the opening vertically, the crucial dimension.

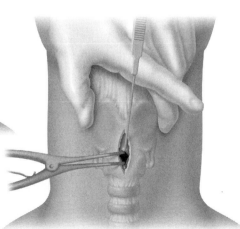

B

8. Insert the Trousseau dilator

The Trousseau dilator may be inserted in one of two ways. One method is to insert the dilator well in through the incision, directing the blades of the dilator longitudinally down the airway. The second method, and the one recommended by the authors, is to insert the dilator minimally into the anterior wound with the blades oriented superiorly and inferiorly, allowing the dilator to open and enlarge the vertical extent of the cricothyroid membrane incision, which is often the anatomically limiting dimension (Fig. 11.7). When this technique is used, care must be taken not to insert the dilator too deeply into the airway, as it will impede subsequent passage of the tracheostomy tube.

9. Insert the tracheostomy tube

The tracheostomy tube, with its inner cannula in situ, is gently inserted through the incision between the blades of the Trousseau dilator. As the tube is advanced gently following its natural curve, the Trousseau dilator is rotated to allow the blades to orient longitudinally in the airway (Fig. 11.8). The tracheostomy tube is advanced until it is firmly seated against the anterior neck. The Trousseau dilator is then removed.

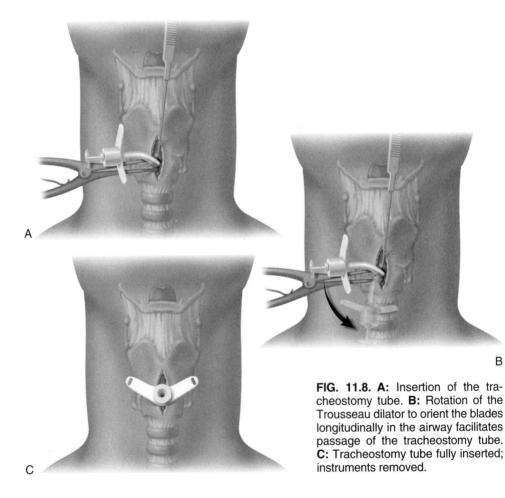

FIG. 11.8. A: Insertion of the tracheostomy tube. **B:** Rotation of the Trousseau dilator to orient the blades longitudinally in the airway facilitates passage of the tracheostomy tube. **C:** Tracheostomy tube fully inserted; instruments removed.

10. Inflate the cuff and confirm tube position

With the cuff inflated, the tracheostomy tube position can be confirmed by the same methods as ETT position. Carbon dioxide detection will reliably indicate correct placement of the tube. If doubt remains, rapid passage of a nasogastric tube through the tracheostomy tube will result in easy passage if the tube is in the trachea and obstruction if the tube has been placed through a false passage into the tissues of the neck. Auscultation of both lungs and the epigastric area is also recommended, although esophageal placement of the tracheostomy tube is exceedingly unlikely. Chest radiography should be performed to assist in the assessment of tube placement and to evaluate for the presence of barotrauma.

B. Success rates and complications

Cricothyrotomy is infrequently performed in emergency departments, so reports of complications are difficult to evaluate. In the National Emergency Airway Registry (NEAR) study, only 1% of more than 4,000 ED intubations involved cricothyrotomy. The most important complication of surgical airway management is failure of the technique, resulting in improper placement or nonplacement of the airway. This is more a failure of technique than a complication and must be recognized immediately, as is the case with a misplaced ETT. Complications such as pneumothorax, significant hemorrhage requiring operative intervention, laryngeal or tracheal injury, and long-term complications, such as subglottic stenosis or permanent voice change, are relatively infrequent and usually minor. The possibility of these complications in no way outweighs the need to establish the airway. In general, the incidence of all complications, both major and minor, is approximately 20%, and most of these complications will be of a minor nature and will not result in long-term morbidity. Box 11.2 lists complications of surgical airway management.

C. Cricothyrotome insertion using the Seldinger technique

Numerous commercial cricothyrotomy devices are available. Several of them utilize a modified Seldinger technique to assist in the placement of a tracheal airway (Fig. 11.9). This method is similar to the one commonly utilized in the placement of central venous catheters and offers some familiarity to the operator uncomfortable or inexperienced with the surgical cricothyrotomy technique described earlier.

  1. *Identification of landmarks.* The cricothyroid membrane is identified by the method described earlier for surgical cricothyrotomy. The nondominant hand is used to control the larynx and maintain identification of the landmarks.

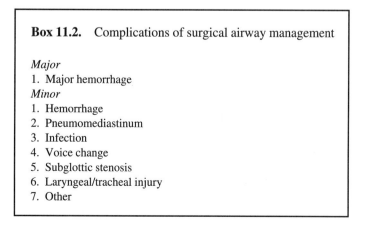

Box 11.2. Complications of surgical airway management

Major
1. Major hemorrhage
Minor
1. Hemorrhage
2. Pneumomediastinum
3. Infection
4. Voice change
5. Subglottic stenosis
6. Laryngeal/tracheal injury
7. Other

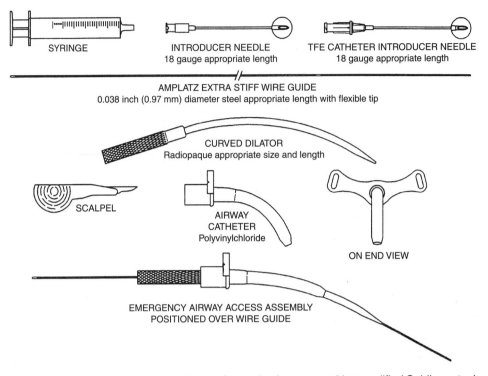

FIG. 11.9. Commercial devices used to perform cricothyrotomy with a modified Seldinger technique. Access is achieved percutaneously through the cricothyroid membrane. The tract is dilated and the airway is established with a 3- to 6-mm-ID tube inserted over the wire guide. (Melker emergency cricothyrotomy catheter sets, Cook Critical Care, Bloomington, IN.)

   2. *Neck preparation.* Antiseptic solution is applied to the anterior neck and, if time permits, infiltration of the site with 1% lidocaine with epinephrine is recommended.
   3. *Locator needle insertion.* The introducer needle (18 gauge) is then inserted into the cricothyroid membrane in a slightly caudal direction. The needle is attached to a syringe and advanced with the dominant hand, while negative pressure is maintained on the syringe. The sudden aspiration of air indicates placement of the needle into the tracheal lumen.
   4. *Guidewire insertion.* The syringe is then removed from the needle. A soft-tipped guidewire is inserted through the needle into the trachea in a caudal direction. The needle is then removed, leaving the wire in place. Control of the wire must be maintained at all times.
   5. *Skin incision.* A small skin incision is then made adjacent to the wire. This facilitates passage of the airway device through the skin. Alternatively, the skin incision may be made vertically over the membrane before insertion of the needle and guidewire.
   6. *Insertion of the airway and dilator.* The airway catheter (3 to 6 mm internal diameter [ID]) with an internal dilator in place is inserted over the wire into the trachea. If resistance is met, the skin incision should be deepened and a gentle twisting motion applied to the airway device. When the airway device is firmly seated in the trachea, the wire and dilator are removed together.

7. *Tube location confirmation.* Tube location can then be confirmed as for surgical cricothyrotomy. The devices are radiopaque on radiographs. The airway must then be secured properly.

III. Direct airway placement devices

Several direct airway devices are commercially available. These generally involve multiple steps in the insertion using a large device that functions as both insertor and airway. The details of the operation of these devices may be obtained from the manufacturer and are provided as inserts with the kits. These devices offer no clear advantage in technique, and they are considered more likely to cause traumatic complications during their insertion than those that employ a Seldinger technique.

IV. Percutaneous transtracheal jet ventilation

Needle cricothyrotomy with percutaneous transtracheal jet ventilation (TTJV) is a surgical airway that may be utilized to temporize in the cannot-intubate, cannot-ventilate situation. Although TTJV is rarely performed in the emergency setting, it is a simple, relatively safe and effective means of ventilation. Advantages of this technique over cricothyrotomy include speed, a simpler technique, and less bleeding. It can also provide an alternative for operators unable to perform a cricothyrotomy. Age is not a contraindication to TTJV, which is the surgical airway of choice for children under 12 years old.

Several other aspects of this technique that differ from cricothyrotomy are important to consider. To provide ventilation, supraglottic patency must be maintained to allow for exhalation. In the case of complete upper-airway obstruction, air stacking from TTJV will cause barotrauma and eventual acidosis; therefore cricothyrotomy is preferable. Another significant difference is that the catheter in TTJV does not provide airway protection. Also, suctioning cannot be adequately performed through the percutaneous catheter. TTJV is therefore best considered a temporizing means of rescue ventilation until a more definitive airway can be obtained.

A. Procedure

1. *Identification of the landmarks.* The anatomy and landmarks used in needle cricothyrotomy are identical to those described earlier for a surgical cricothyrotomy. If there are no contraindications, the head of the patient should be extended. Placing a towel under the shoulders may facilitate cervical hyperextension. The area overlying the cricothyroid membrane should be prepared with an antiseptic solution and, if time permits, anesthetized with 1% lidocaine and epinephrine.

2. *Immobilize the larynx.* Use the thumb and the middle fingers of the nondominant hand to stabilize the larynx and cricoid cartilage while the index finger palpates the cricothyroid membrane (Fig. 11.10A). It is essential to maintain control of the larynx throughout the procedure.

3. *Transtracheal needle insertion.* A large-bore intravenous catheter (12 to 16 gauge) is attached to a 20-ml syringe, which may be empty or partially filled with a clear liquid. A 15-degree angle can be placed 2.5 cm from the distal end of the intravenous catheter or a commercially available catheter can be employed (see "Equipment" later). The dominant hand holds the syringe with the needle directed caudally in the long axis of the trachea at a 30-degree angle to the skin (Fig. 11.10B). While maintaining negative pressure on the syringe, the needle is inserted through the cricothyroid membrane into the trachea. As soon as the needle enters the trachea, the syringe will easily fill with air. If a liquid is used bubbles will appear. Any resistance implies that the catheter remains in the tissue. In the awake patient, lidocaine may be used in the syringe and then injected into the tracheal lumen to suppress the cough reflex.

4. *Catheter advancement.* Once entry into the trachea is confirmed, the catheter can be advanced. The needle may be partially or completely withdrawn before advancement;

however, the needle should not be advanced with the catheter (Fig. 11.10C). A small incision can assist with catheter advancement if there is resistance at the skin.

5. *Confirmation of location.* The catheter should be advanced to the hub and controlled by hand at all times. Air should be reaspirated to confirm once again the location of the catheter within the trachea (Fig. 11.10D,E).

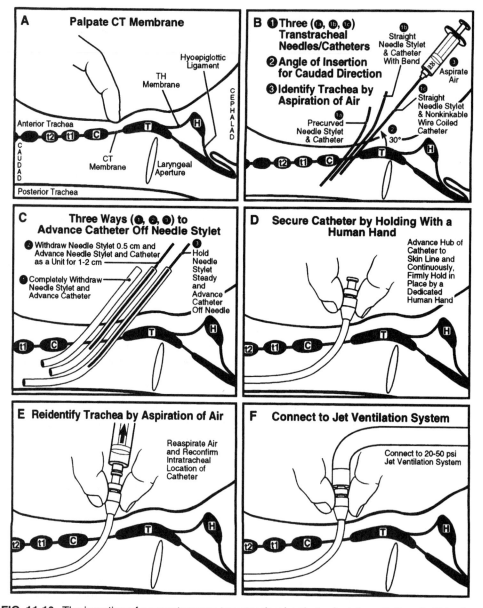

FIG. 11.10. The insertion of a percutaneous transtracheal catheter for jet ventilation. **A:** Cricothyroid membrane is identified and the larynx is controlled. **B:** Needle catheter is inserted percutaneously. **C:** Catheter is advanced. **D:** Catheter must be secured at all times by hand. **E:** Intratracheal location is reconfirmed. **F:** Connection to a jet ventilation system. (Abbreviations: T, thyroid cartilage; H, hyoid bone; C, cricoid cartilage; t1, first tracheal cartilage.) (Adapted from Benumof JL. Trans-tracheal jet ventilation via percutaneous catheter and high-pressure source. In: Benumof JL, ed. *Airway management: principles and practice.* St Louis: Mosby, 1996.)

6. *Connection to jet ventilation.* The catheter is then connected to the female end of the polyvinyl chloride (PVC) tubing of the jet ventilation system by a luer lock. The hub should not be secured in place by anything other than a human hand until a definitive airway is established. Firm, constant pressure must be applied by hand to ensure that proper positioning is maintained and to create a seal at the skin to minimize air leak.

7. *Technique of jet ventilation.* In the adult, the jet ventilation system should be connected to an oxygen source of 50 pounds per square inch (psi). In general, inspiration is less than 1 second followed by 2 to 3 seconds of expiration. Since the gas flow through a 14-gauge needle at 50 psi is 1,600 ml/sec, less than 1 second of inspiratory time is required for an adequate tidal volume in a normally compliant lung. Exhalation depends on the elastic recoil of the lung, which is a relatively low driving pressure. Therefore the recommended inspiratory-to-expiratory ratio (I : E) is 1 : 3. It is very important to maintain upper-airway patency to allow for exhalation and avoid air trapping and barotrauma. All patients should have an oral and nasal airway placed. For small adults and children, oxygen pressure should be down-regulated to 20 to 30 psi if possible. For children under 5, a bag should be used for ventilation.

B. Equipment

1. Transtracheal catheters

   A large-bore intravenous catheter is acceptable. The proper placement is made easier by placing a small angle 2.5 cm from the tip. Commercially available devices include precurved (Acutronic, Germany) and nonkinkable wire-coiled (Cook Critical Care, Bloomington, IN) catheters (Fig. 11.11). The wire-coiled catheter will not link when bent, therefore providing a more secure airway.

2. Transtracheal jet ventilation systems

   The TTJV system consists of a high-pressure oxygen source (usually central wall-oxygen pressure of 50 psi); high-pressure oxygen tubing; an on/off valve to control inspiration; high-pressure PVC tubing; and a luer lock to connect to the catheter (Fig. 11.12).

   A regulator to control the maximal pressure is optional but highly recommended. This is particularly useful where barotrauma is a concern and in pediatrics, where the inspiratory pressures should be lowered to 20 to 30 psi. Although a system can be assembled inexpensively from readily available materials, a commercially made, preassembled system is recommended. The quality assurance when it is required is worth the marginal increase in cost.

   A TTJV system can also be connected to a low-flow portable oxygen tank when circumstances require mobility. When the flow is set at the maximal 15 L/min and no flow is allowed, the pressure temporarily increases to 120 psi. Once flow is released, high flow occurs momentarily and then rapidly decreases to the steady state of 5 to 10 psi. Adequate tidal volumes may be achieved through a 14-gauge catheter in the first 0.5 second. A shorter I : E ratio of 1 : 1 is recommended.

   Another setup using manual ventilation with a self-inflating reservoir bag has been described utilizing standard equipment found in any emergency department. Bag ventilation may be connected directly to the percutaneous transtracheal

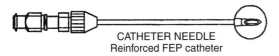

CATHETER NEEDLE
Reinforced FEP catheter

FIG. 11.11. Nonkinkable wire-coiled transtracheal jet ventilation catheter. (Cook Critical Care, Bloomington, IN.)

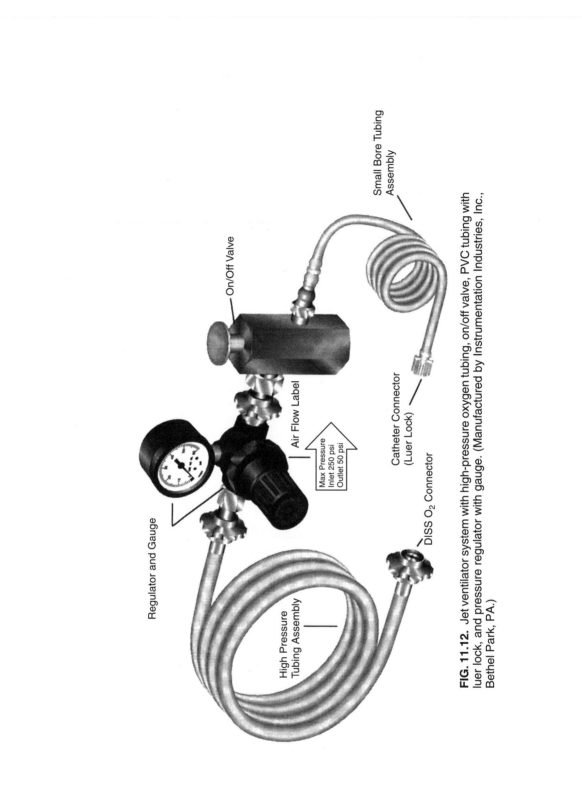

Small Bore Tubing
Assembly

On/Off Valve

Catheter Connector
(Luer Lock)

Air Flow Label

Max Pressure
Inlet 250 psi
Outlet 50 psi

DISS O$_2$ Connector

Regulator and Gauge

High Pressure
Tubing Assembly

FIG. 11.12. Jet ventilator system with high-pressure oxygen tubing, on/off valve, PVC tubing with luer lock, and pressure regulator with gauge. (Manufactured by Instrumentation Industries, Inc., Bethel Park, PA.)

catheter in two ways. The male end of a 15-mm ETT adapter from a 3-mm-ID ETT will fit directly into the catheter. Alternatively, the male end of a plungerless 3-ml syringe will fit into the catheter and the male end of an 8-mm-ID ETT adapter will then insert into the female end of the empty syringe. Ventilation is temporary at best and P_aCO_2 will increase at a rate of 4 mmHg/min. Even the simple assembly of this system is too time-consuming to be done during the event, so it must be pre-assembled. This may have utility in the pediatric patient less than 5 years old when a regulator to control inspiratory pressures is unavailable. In general, children under 5 years old should receive TTJV via a ventilation bag; age 5 to 12 years old at 30 mmHg and >12 years to adult at 30 to 50 mmHg. A catheter of less than 3 mm ID will be insufficient to adequately ventilate/oxygenate the adult patient using a bag, and 50 psi oxygen is required.

C. Complications specific to TTJV

- Subcutaneous emphysema
- Barotrauma
- Reflex cough with each ventilation (may be aborted with lidocaine)
- Catheter kinking
- Obstruction from blood or mucus
- Esophageal puncture
- Mucosal damage if nonhumidified gas is used

V. Tips and pearls

Surgical airway management is rarely the method of first choice for patients in the emergency department. However, there is a population of patients for whom surgical airway management will literally make the difference between life and death. Therefore emergency physicians must be proficient with surgical airway management.

There may be little advantage to using a cricothyrotome rather than a formal, surgical cricothyroidotomy set. Time of performance of the procedure, complication rates, degree of difficulty, and success rates are all comparable between the two methods. Of the available cricothyrotomes, those that use the Seldinger technique are preferable. Personal preference should guide selection. There is no evidence that any cricothyrotome can successfully be placed in a child under 10 to 12 years of age, regardless of the design of the device or the claims of the manufacturer.

Percutaneous transtracheal ventilation is virtually never indicated in the adult patient. In adults, establishment of a more functional surgical airway using a cricothyrotome or by formal cricothyroidotomy is vastly preferable. However, percutaneous transtracheal ventilation remains a useful temporizing measure. In children under 12, the opposite is true. In this age group, percutaneous transtracheal ventilation is the primary surgical airway management method of choice and cricothyrotomy and cricothyrotomes should be avoided. Despite the extreme infrequency of use of percutaneous transtracheal ventilation in the emergency department, it is important to have a percutaneous transtracheal ventilation set readily available and to be familiar with how to connect and use it. The wire-coiled catheter designed for TTJV is preferable to standard IV catheters because of the tendency for the latter to kink.

Of the methods described in this chapter, only a formal surgical cricothyroidotomy results in the placement of a cuffed tube within the trachea. All the other techniques described here must be considered temporary at best. Placement of a tracheostomy or ETT through a formal surgical cricothyrotomy incision results in an airway that can be used as a definitive airway for the patient, if desired.

The #4 Shiley cuffed tracheostomy tube, which has an inside diameter of 5 mm, should be used for virtually all cases of adult cricothyrotomy in the emergency department. The tube is of adequate size to provide ventilation in virtually all circumstances, and its outside dimensions are such that it will almost always be easily inserted. For very large adult men, a #6 Shiley can be used.

ADDITIONAL READING

Benumof JL. Trans-tracheal jet ventilation via percutaneous catheter and high-pressure source. In: Benumof JL, ed. *Airway management: principles and practice.* St Louis: Mosby, 1996.

Benumof JL, Scheller MS. The importance of transtracheal jet ventilation in the management of the difficult airway. *Anesthesiology* 1989;71:769.

Burkey B, Esclamado R, Morganroth M. The role of cricothyroidotomy in airway management. *Clin Chest Med* 1991;12:561–571.

DeLaurier GA, Hawkins ML, Treat RC, et al. Acute airway management: role of cricothyroidotomy. *Am Surg* 1990;56:12–15.

Egol A, Culpepper JA, Snyder JV. Barotrauma and hypotension resulting from jet ventilation in critically ill patients. *Chest* 1985;88:98.

Jacobson LE, Gomez GA, Sobieray RJ, et al. Surgical cricothyroidotomy in trauma patients: analysis of its use by paramedics in the field. *J Trauma* 1996;41:15–20.

Leibovici D, Fredman B, Gofrit ON, et al. Prehospital cricothyroidotomy by physicians. *Am J Emerg Med* 1997; 15:91–93.

Salvino CK, Dries D, Gamelli R, et al. Emergency cricothyroidotomy in trauma victims. *J Trauma* 1993;34:503–505.

Walls RM. Cricothyroidotomy In: Campbell WH, ed. *Emergency medicine clinics of North America.* Philadelphia: WB Saunders, 1988.

12

Pediatric Airway Techniques

Robert C. Luten

Professor of Emergency Medicine and Pediatrics,
University of Florida, Jacksonville, Florida

In general, all the airway techniques used in adults can be used in large or older children (adolescents). Few of these techniques, however, are appropriate for infants (<1 year) and small children (<3 years). This is because of the smaller size and configuration of the young airway that precludes their utility.

The following techniques are used in infants and small children and will be briefly reviewed or referenced:

Basic: Bag valve mask (BVM) ventilation
           Endotracheal intubation
Advanced: Laryngeal mask
           Lightwand
           Needle cricothyroidotomy

The following techniques used in older children (>10 years old) and adults but *not* used in small children (infrequently if <10 years, never if <3 years old) include:

Blind nasotracheal intubation
Combitube
Surgical cricothyroidotomy (never under 10 years of age)

I. Basic techniques: BVM ventilation and endotracheal intubation

These techniques are both reviewed thoroughly in this manual. The use of oral and naso-pharyngeal airways, frequent adjuncts to BVM ventilation, is important. The rationale for the use of specific equipment (curved or straight blades, cuffed versus uncuffed tubes) is described in Chapter 17. As opposed to airway management in adults, unless one has size-appropriate equipment, the procedure will be doomed to failure, even in the most experienced hands.

The importance of good BVM technique in advanced airway management cannot be overemphasized. Although standard rapid sequence intubation optimally requires none, BVM ventilation with simultaneous cricoid pressure is frequently needed to buy time in hypoxemic pediatric patients until optimal intubation conditions can be achieved. Comfort with manipulation (positioning) of the airway, smaller tidal volumes, and specific equipment is essential. A list of tips for successful BVM ventilation and endotracheal intubation is provided later.

A. Tips for successful BVM and endotracheal intubation in infants and children

    1. Positioning

        Proper positioning is the key to successful BVM as well as endotracheal intubation. Children have a relatively large occiput compared with adults. In the supine position, the occiput of the unsupported relaxed patient may cause flexion of the head and neck and resultant airway obstruction. Proper positioning of the patient is key to prevent obstruction and provide optimal alignment of the axes of the airway (Chapter 17). Optimal alignment of the laryngeal, pharyngeal, and oral axes in adults usually requires elevation of the occiput to flex the neck on the torso and *hyperextension* of the head at the atlantooccipital joint. Because of the larger relative size of the occiput in children, elevation of the occiput is unnecessary and *hyperextension* of the head may actually cause obstruction. Slight anterior displacement of the atlantooccipital junction is all that is needed (pulling up on the chin to create the "sniffing" position). Normally, support of the resultant anatomic alignment with a towel between the head and shoulders to prevent flexion of the neck on the chest in the relaxed patient is all that is necessary. On rare occasions, elevation of the shoulders in the small infant may be needed to counteract the effect of the large occiput that causes the head to flex forward to the chest. These are guidelines only. Each individual patient is different. A quick trial of the "most commonly successful" and even the "potentially helpful" positions to find the optimal position for your patient may be warranted (Fig. 12.1A, C).

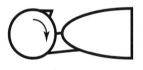

Flexion of the head on the chest in the unsupported, relaxed, supine patient potentially causing airway obstruction.

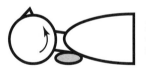

Normal supine alignment with slight extension of the head at the Atlanto-occipital junction by pulling the chin to the "sniffing" position. Support of this alignment with a towel roll between the head and shoulders.

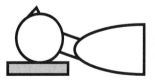

Hyperextension of the head at the Alanto-occipital junction. Commonly used in adolescents and adults, occasionally in children.

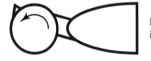

Elevation of the occiput to flex the neck on the torso. Commonly used in adolescents and adults, occasionally in children.

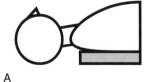

Elevation of the shoulders. On rare occasions helpful in newborns and small infants only. Can potentially obstruct the airway of older children and adults.

A

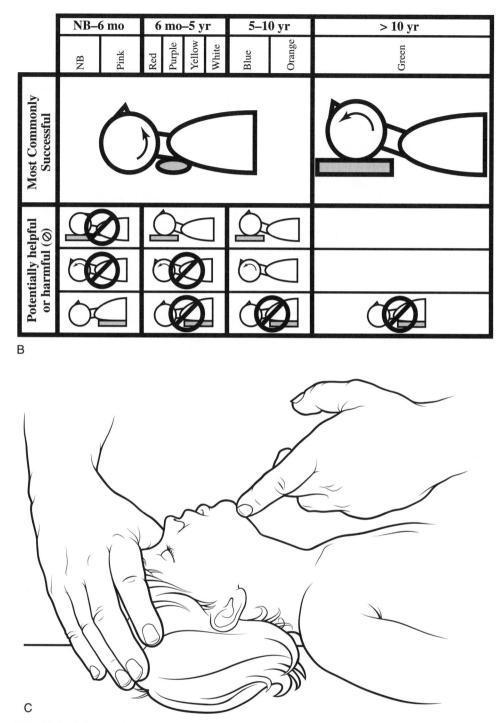

	NB–6 mo		6 mo–5 yr				5–10 yr		> 10 yr
	NB	Pink	Red	Purple	Yellow	White	Blue	Orange	Green

FIG. 12.1. A,B: Positioning. Proper positioning is the key to successful bag-and-mask ventilation as well as endotracheal intubation. Children have a relatively large occiput compared with adults. Proper positioning of the patient is key to prevent obstruction and provide optimal alignment of the axes of the airway. Optimal alignment of the laryngeal, pharyngeal, and oral axes in adults usually requires elevation of the occiput to flex the neck on the torso and hyperextension of the head at the atlantooccipital joint. (See text for details.) **C:** For most children simply extending the patient's head on the atlantooccipital joint by elevating the chin is all that is required for optimal airway axis alignment and patency. Quick trial and error for optimal position (**A,B**) may be necessary.

2. Bag-and-mask ventilation (BMV)

The previously described positioning is usually obtained simultaneously while applying the one-handed "C-grip" technique. The thumb and forefinger place and support the mask from the bridge of the nose to the cleft of the chin, avoiding the eyes. The bony prominences of the chin are lifted up by the rest of fingers, placing the head in mild extension to form the sniffing position. Care is taken to avoid pressure on the airway anteriorly to avoid collapsing and obstructing the pliable trachea. The cadence for bagging can be facilitated by the mnemonic "squeeze, release, release," which will allow adequate time for exhalation during the cycle. If ventilation is not immediately obtained with these maneuvers, an oral airway should be inserted to lift the tongue off the posterior pharynx, the most common site of obstruction.

3. Endotracheal intubation

Once positioning has been attempted, further manipulation of the airway may increase visualization (e.g., pressure on the thyroid cartilage to move the glottis opening into the laryngoscopic view).

4. BMV and cricoid pressure

It is essential to master BMV and cricoid pressure in both adults and children to provide longer protected time from hypoxia. Studies in children have shown that cricoid pressure not only prevents passive regurgitation, but also prevents gastric insufflation, even with ventilation pressures greater than 40 cm H_2O. This is especially important in infants, in whom gastric distention leads to decreased respiratory excursion and increases the chances of aspiration.

5. Pop-off valves help and harm

A pop-off valve is designed to prevent the delivery of excessive volume, and therefore, excessive pressure, to the lungs. At a preset level, an escape valve opens and keeps the pressure below dangerous levels, usually <40 cm H_2O. However, certain conditions require higher pressures to overcome upper-airway obstruction or to open noncompliant lungs—in these situations occlude the valve manually or with the built-in occluding device. Remember, before diagnosing elevated compliance, exclude inadequate airway patency as the cause; that is, manipulate the airway position to optimize patency.

6. Clinical confirmation of adequate tidal volume

Although infants differ in size and therefore tidal volumes, a length-based measurement can give adequate starting tidal volumes. However, they are just that: starting volumes. Always assess adequacy by careful examination for chest wall rise, increasing volumes as necessary.

II. Advanced techniques

A. Laryngeal masks

The use of the laryngeal mask airway (LMA) as an alternative airway is reviewed in Chapter 5. Its use in the pediatric patient is well described and was recently reviewed (Tobias, *Pediatr Emerg Care* 1996;12:370). Many difficult airway carts contain an LMA, which is particularly useful in superior, anterior airways. Since most normal small pediatric airways are superior and anteriorly positioned, it would seem logical that the LMA would be a viable airway alternative in children. The airway comes in various sizes, and facility with size will be taught in the skill stations.

B. Pediatric lightwand

The lightwand is discussed elsewhere. Recently, fiberoptic intubation stylets have been marketed for children. Although experience with these devices is limited in children, relative ease of use and a low complication rate make the lighted stylet a viable airway alternative in the relatively stable patient.

C. Needle cricothyroidotomy

Every textbook chapter, article, or lecture on pediatric airway management refers to the technique of needle cricothyroidotomy as the recommended last-resort rescue procedure. This is the case despite the fact that there is little literature to support its use and safety, and the fact that hardly any of the "experts" who write about needle cricothyroidotomy have significant experience performing the procedure on a live human patient. Nevertheless, any clinician who manages pediatric emergencies as part of his or her practice must be familiar with the procedure and its indications, and have the appropriate equipment readily accessible in the emergency department.

Needle cricothyroidotomy is indicated as a life-saving, last-resort procedure in patients who present or progress to the "cannot intubate, cannot ventilate" scenario and whose obstruction is proximal to glottic opening. The classic indication is epiglottitis where BVM ventilation and intubation have failed. Other indications include facial trauma, angioedema, and other conditions that preclude proximal access to the glottic opening. Needle cricothyroidotomy is rarely helpful in patients who have aspirated a foreign body that cannot be visualized by direct laryngoscopy, as it is unlikely that the obstruction is located proximal to the cricothyroid membrane. It also would be of questionable value in the patient with croup, as the obstruction is subglottic, and more likely to be bypassed by an endotracheal tube (ETT) introduced orally into the trachea with a stylet, rather than blindly by needle cricothyroidotomy.

1. Equipment

Various premade kits have been recommended for percutaneous needle cricothyrotomy. These kits are not recommended in infants and small children. The simplest equipment, appropriate for use in infants, consists of the following:

14-gauge over-the-needle catheter

3.0-mm ETT adapter

5-ml syringe

It is a good practice to preassemble the kit, place it in a sealed, clear bag, and tape it in an accessible position in the resuscitation area.

2. Procedure

Place the child in the supine position with the head extended. Place a towel under the shoulder to further exaggerate the extension. This forces the trachea anteriorly so that it becomes easily palpable and can be stabilized with two fingers of one hand. The following statement appears in all textbooks describing this procedure: "Carefully palpate the cricothyroid membrane." In reality it is very difficult to do this in an infant. If you cannot palpate the membrane, you should still proceed. The priority is an airway and provision of oxygen. Complications from inserting the catheter elsewhere into the trachea besides the cricothyroid membrane can be addressed later. Consider the trachea as a large vein, and cannulate it with your catheter directed caudally. Attach the 3.0-mm ETT adapter and a ventilation bag with oxygen at flush; commence bag ventilation. Studies in canine models demonstrate adequate oxygenation can be obtained in subjects with a weight of up to 30 kg, which is equivalent to the weight of a 10-year-old child. The provider will note exaggerated resistance to bagging. This is normal and is related to the turbulence created by using a 14-gauge catheter as an airway and is not the result of a misplaced catheter or poor lung compliance secondary to pneumothorax. It is helpful to practice BVM ventilation through a catheter to experience the feel of the significantly increased resistance. Jet ventilation has also been advocated in this situation. Extreme caution, however, must be exercised to avoid the complications of excessive flow and resultant barotrauma. Jet ventilation should only be considered by those experienced in its use and in children more than 5 to 6 years old. Even in a child of 6 or older, if adequate oxygen saturation can be maintained with the bag technique described previously, this is preferable to jet ventilation. If jet ventilation is used, start with low psi (20 mmHg) and titrate to adequate chest rise and fall and oxygen saturation.

III. Procedures used in adolescents and adults but not in small children.

A. Blind nasotracheal intubation

Nasotracheal intubation in children is uniformly discouraged and is frequently considered contraindicated in children. This recommendation is based on the fact that the sharp angle of the nasopharynx and pharyngotracheal axis in children precludes a high percentage of success with this technique when performed blindly. A second reason is that children are at increased risk for hemorrhage because of preponderance of highly vascular and delicate adenoidal tissue. The direct-visualization technique is, however, commonly used in small infants and children. Aided by direct visualization with a laryngoscope once the ETT has passed into the oro- and hypopharynx, tracheal placement is aided with Magill forceps. However, this technique is not helpful in emergency airway management. In general, the technique of blind nasotracheal intubation, which is essentially the same as that described for adults in Chapter 8, is not recommended below 10 years of age.

B. Combitube

The Combitube represents an excellent, easily learned alternative that is not yet available for pediatric use. However, there is no reason a large child or adolescent more than 4 feet tall would not be an anatomically appropriate subject for its application. The use of the Combitube is described elsewhere in this manual.

C. Surgical cricothyroidotomy

The cricothyroid membrane in small infants and children is minimally developed (Fig. 12.2). Identification of the key landmarks is at best extremely difficult, even in the noncrisis situation. The complication rate from attempts to perform this procedure in an emergency precludes its use as a recommended alternative in pediatric ad-

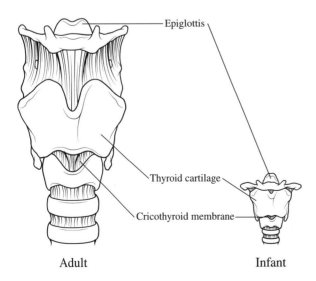

Adult   Infant

FIG. 12.2. Cricothyroid membrane. Comparative size of the adult (**LEFT**) versus pediatric (**RIGHT**) cricothyroid membrane. Note that not only is the larynx smaller, but the actual membrane is smaller proportionately in comparison involving $1/4$ to $1/3$ the anterior tracheal circumference versus $2/3$ to $3/4$ in the adult. This pediatric drawing is that of a toddler, which accommodates a 4.5-mm ETT.

vanced airway management. As with adults, adolescents may have easily identifiable and accessible anatomy, therefore this procedure is recommended in this age group as is transtracheal ventilation. Cricothyroidotomy using a commercially available kit (Pedi-trake) has *not* been shown to be successful or even safe. Surgical or cricothyrotome-based cricothyrotomy should not be attempted in children under 10, except in extraordinary circumstances. In children under 10 years of age, needle cricothyrotomy with bag or jet ventilation is preferable.

IV. **Summary recommendations for invasive airway procedures in children:**
<5 years old
Needle cricothyrotomy and bag ventilation
> Equipment: 14 gauge catheter
> 3.0 ETT adapter
> BVM
> 5-ml syringe

5 to 10 years old
Needle cricothyrotomy and bag ventilation
If unsuccessful, options include:
> a. Use of dilator (4-mm ID) from Melker cricothyrotome kit to convert to tracheostomy tube
> b. TTJV regulated to low psi
> adapted to 14F gauge catheter

>10 years
> Operator preference
> Cricothyrotome with bag ventilation
> or
> Surgical cricothyrotomy
> or
> Needle cricothyrotomy with TTJV

ADDITIONAL READING

Dickinson AE. The normal and abnormal pediatric upper airway: recognition and management of obstruction. *Clin Chest Med* 1987;8:583–596.

Dobbinson, TL, Whalen J, Pelton DA, et al. Needle tracheostomy: a laboratory study. *Anaesth Intensive Care* 1980;8:72–80.

Fanconi S, Dangel P. Cuffed tubes in pediatric patients. *Crit Care Med* 1987;15:626–627.

Klein E, Quan L. Neonatal resuscitation. In: Rosen P, Barkin R, Danzl D, et al., eds. *Emergency medicine: concepts and clinical practice,* 4th ed. St Louis: Mosby, 1998.

Mellick LB, Dierking BH. One size doesn't fit all: choosing pediatric equipment, part II. *J Emerg Med Serv* 1991;17:35–46.

Moynihan RJ, Brock-Utne JG, Archer JC, et al. The effect of cricoid pressure on preventing gastric insufflation in infants and children. *Anesthesiology* 1993;78:652–656.

Reich DL, Mingus M. Transtracheal oxygenation using simple equipment and a low-pressure oxygen source. *Crit Care Med* 1990;18:664–665.

Tobias JD. Laryngeal mask airway: a review for the emergency physician. *Pediatr Emerg Care* 1996;12:370–377.

Zaritsky A, Luten RC. Pediatric resuscitation. In: Rosen P, Barkin R, Danzl D, et al., eds. *Emergency medicine: concepts and clinical practice,* 4th ed. St Louis: Mosby, 1998.

13

The Difficult Airway in Pediatrics

Robert C. Luten

Professor of Emergency Medicine and Pediatrics,
University of Florida, Jacksonville, Florida

Securing an airway in a patient, adult or child, is made more challenging or "difficult" for two principal reasons:

1. The patient's normal airway anatomy is modified because of an acute insult or
2. A patient with an abnormal airway (e.g., a congenital anomaly) requires airway management for an unrelated cause, such as respiratory failure due to an asthma exacerbation.

There are contributing factors related to pediatric airway management that intensify the challenge, thus the difficulty of managing emergent airways. The approach to the emergent difficult adult airways is well described in this manual. Pediatric difficult airways, especially those encountered in emergency situations, are far less common, not well studied, and not extensively covered in any textbook. This chapter attempts to put in perspective the issues and problems related to pediatric airway management so that the clinician can become more comfortable and competent when managing them. For purposes of this discussion, difficult pediatric airways will be divided functionally into difficult airways secondary to

1. Normal anatomic differences from the adult airway and relative infrequency of encountering the pediatric airway
2. Acute infectious disease
3. Acute noninfectious disease
4. Congenital anomalies, most commonly with a superimposed indication for emergent airway management unrelated to the airway abnormality (e.g., respiratory failure secondary to asthma or pneumonia). Most of the airway/anesthesia literature and textbooks cover the topic of airway management of congenital anomalies. However, this is usually done in the context of the stable patient undergoing elective surgery, and these patients are managed by experienced subspecialists. This information is therefore of limited value to the practicing emergency physician.

I. The difficult airway secondary to anatomic differences and unfamiliarity

Effective emergency airway management requires rapid evaluation, decision making, and treatment. The amount of time that is required to do this is finite. In any situation, the human mind has limited ability for what is called "critical thinking"—the essential skill in evaluating and prioritizing information in an emergency and arriving at an optimal and practical strategy. In adult emergencies the emergency physician familiar with adult drug doses, equipment sizes, and normal vital signs is free to maximize his or her patient contact time for critical thinking. In a pediatric emergency the large variation in size causes lack of familiarity with equipment sizes, drug doses, and other related parameters. Clinicians are not free from consideration of all these extraneous variables during patient encounters; therefore their time is occupied with these issues and they cannot maximize "critical thinking" time (i.e., concentrate on the priorities of airway management). The color-coded, Broselow-Luten, length-based emergency system referred to in Chapter 17 is one way to eliminate these age- and size-related variables from consideration during the crisis, thus permitting the emergency physicians to concentrate on priorities only.

The pediatric airway, especially in the first 2 to 3 years of life, is different from the adult airway. These differences are outlined in Chapter 17. It is not that these differences alone make it more difficult to manage, but that they are so infrequently encountered in clinical practice that they can become a barrier if one is not aware of them on an ongoing basis.

If one looks at any major textbook in emergency medicine or pediatric emergency medicine, one will find procedures, strategies, and recommendations suggested as if they are commonly used and therefore should be part of the armamentarium of the practicing emergency physician, when in fact they are not. An example is needle cricothyroidotomy in a young infant. Few authors themselves have experience with this technique, and it has not been studied in emergency clinical situations. This type of information must be put in perspective for the practicing emergency physician and he or she should be given practical alternatives, useful in real situations. In summary, a series of differences and non-focused information conspire to make the management of the emergent pediatric airway challenging for the emergency physician. In fact, most of these anatomic differences require only modest, commonsense adjustments to technique, and the principles of pediatric airway management mirror those for the adult airway.

II. Difficult airways secondary to acute infectious disease

1. Epiglottitis
2. Croup (usually not a difficult intubation; see Table 13.1)
3. Retropharyngeal abscess
4. Bacterial tracheitis
5. Ludwig's angina

Most of the entities in this and the next section present because the normal anatomy is altered, usually by swelling, which leads to varying degrees of airway obstruction.

The pediatric patient is especially susceptible to airway obstruction from swelling, often from conditions that are less threatening to the adult. This is illustrated in Box 13.1, which outlines the effect of 1-mm edema on airway resistance in the infant (4-mm airway diameter) versus adult (8-mm airway diameter).

It should also be noted that these figures reflect the quietly breathing infant or adult. The crying child increases the work of breathing 32-fold, hence the principle of maintaining children in a quiet, comfortable environment during evaluation and management for potential airway obstruction.

Table 13.1 outlines the two most commonly referred to infectious diseases involving the upper airway with potential for obstruction in children (epiglottitis and croup) as well as the management of one of the most feared noninfectious airway problems, foreign-body aspiration. The reality is that epiglottitis is rarely seen since the introduction of the *Hemophilus influenzae* vaccine, and croup, commonly referred to in the differential diagnosis of epiglottitis, is usually a clinically distinct entity and is even more rarely a difficult intubation, as the obstruction is subglottic. It is of value still to discuss epiglottitis because

TABLE 13.1. *Management of the "most–feared" pediatrics airway problems*

Disease	Pathology and deterioration	Approach	FB removal maneuvers	BVM two person techniques	Intubation	Needle cricothyrotomy
Epiglottitis	Rapidly progressing disease process affecting the supraglottic structures (epiglottis, aryepiglottic folds). Patients usually present in minimal distress. Decompensation rarely occurs unless the patient is overstimulated or manipulated, leading to increasing airway resistance or functional obstruction. Otherwise, decompensation is the result of progressive deterioration over time secondary to fatigue, although the respiratory arrest may occur precipitously.	Stable → observe → transfer to O.R. for definitive airway Decompensation BVM ↓ Intubation ↓ Needle cric	Not indicated	Effective in *most* patients who deteriorate. Technique: 2-handed seal with another rescuer providing sufficient pressure to Overcome the obstruction	Usually successful. Use tube size 1 mm smaller. Use stylet. Suction, visualize, press on chest and look for bubble.	Probably one of the few indications for needle cric *if* BMV *and* intubation unsuccessful
Croup	Slowly progressive (hours to days) disease process affecting the subglottic trachea, causing dynamic inspiratory augmented obstruction. Deterioration is usually progressive rather than sudden and related to respiratory muscle fatigue, and as in the case of epiglottis, the arrest may also occur precipitously.	Racemic epi Steroids Stable → ICU Decompensation ↓ BMV ↓ Intubation	Not indicated	Effective. Positive pressure overcomes obstruction by acting as a stent. Will also probably require higher pressures.	Proximal airway normal; therefore should not be problematic. Consider ET tube 1 size smaller and use stylet.	Not indicated since obstruction is distal
FB aspiration	Patients with aspirated foreign bodies continuously have the potential for decompensation secondary to acute airway obstruction. The level of obstruction may vary from the hypopharynx, above or below the glottis, to the mainstem bronchus.	Stable → observe → transfer for removal Decompensation: Direct visualization and removal with Magill ↓ FB removal maneuvers ↓ Intubation to force FB distally into mainstem bronchus	Indicated if *appropriate* only 1. Patient clinically obstructed 2. Direct visualization and removal attempted if equipment available	Should not be used prior to attempts to remove FB. May be obviated by intubation.	Last resort in an effort to push FB distally.	Not indicated since FB will be distal to the obstruction if other efforts have failed.

Abbreviations: BVM, bag, valve, mask; FB, foreign body; epi, epinephrine; ICU, intensive care unit; OR, operating room.

Box 13.1

	Change in cross-sectional area	Change in resistance
Infant	44% decrease	200% increase
Adult	25% decrease	40% increase

it represents the prototype indication for needle cricothyrotomy (Chapter 11) for obstruction proximal to the glottic opening when bag-valve-mask (BVM) ventilation and intubation fail. Other problems causing obstruction proximal to the glottic opening include facial trauma, angioedema, and caustic ingestions and burns involving the hypopharynx. To put these "most-feared" diseases in perspective, the following points should be kept in mind:

1. All these problems have in common the fact that airway intervention should never be attempted unless deterioration occurs or is imminent. If one adheres to this principle and then follows a stepwise approach as outlined in Table 13.1, results will be optimal and complications, especially iatrogenic complications, will be avoided.

2. Epiglottitis and croup are *clinically very distinct entities,* rarely, if ever, requiring an x-ray to distinguish the two. The fact that textbooks group them together in the differential diagnosis of acute life-threatening upper-airway obstruction is misleading, as the differentiation is usually clinically obvious.

3. Croup, as opposed to epiglottitis or foreign-body aspiration, will respond to *medical intervention* (inhaled epinephrine), thus usually avoiding the need for intubation.

4. Retropharyngeal abscess in children *usually presents without airway compromise,* although it is virtually always found in textbooks in the differential diagnosis of acute life-threatening airway obstruction. The same is true of Ludwig's angina, an even less common disease. These diseases will be referred to in the next section as "paraairway involvement" diseases for this reason.

III. **Difficult airways secondary to noninfectious causes**
   1. Foreign body
   2. Burns
   3. Anaphylaxis
   4. Caustic ingestion
   5. Trauma
   6. Other swellings (angioneurotic edema, Quinke's disease, etc.)

Foreign-body aspiration is probably the most feared pediatric airway problem. Aspirated foreign bodies account for significant mortality in the infant and toddler age group. As opposed to other airway entities, a plan of expectant observation until definitive management by preestablished protocol involving consultants is usually recommended (Table 13.1). Intervention should only be attempted if total obstruction occurs. Otherwise, extraction is best achieved in a controlled environment with standby surgical backup present.

Table 13.2 discusses timing of airway intervention and groups entities from both infectious and noninfectious causes according to timing of intervention. A knowledge of the signs and symptoms of impending airway obstruction in children is key to the approach to the early intervention group (group B) diseases that, if left to expectant treatment, have a greater potential for deterioration. An example is the burn or anaphylaxis patient unresponsive to management who is beginning to develop a raspy voice.

Group A represents patients whose airway should be actively managed in the emergency department (ED) only if deterioration occurs. The rationale in these cases is that

TABLE 13.2. *Timing of intervention*

Group A. Intervene *only* if deterioration occurs
        Foreign body
        Para-airway diagnoses* (diseases such as retropharyngeal or peritonillar
          abscess or Ludwig's angina that are usually stable on presentation and
          deterioration is uncommon)
        Epiglottitis
        Croup (not really difficult intubation, in the sense that visualization of this
          airway by laryngoscopy is relatively unaffected)

Group B. Intervene *early* (preventively)
        Burns
        Anaphylaxis (usually responds to medical treatment)
        Caustic ingestions
        Trauma

* These are disease entities that present to the emergency department (ED). They involve infection and swelling proximal to the tracheal opening. Diagnosis can be made clinically or confirmed with imaging studies, but these conditions rarely require emergent intervention. Provisions for definitive airway management must be in place; however, the majority of these patients do not require it and respond to medical (antibiotics) or surgical management. Unfortunately, these entities are included in textbooks under the differential diagnosis for airway obstruction, creating the false impression that deterioration is a common occurrence, requesting ED intervention.

intervention is best done in controlled circumstances by a multidisciplinary team of experienced operators. Treatment in less than ideal conditions may lead to untoward outcomes. An example is the child with an aspirated foreign body. This patient is best served by transportation to the operating room (OR) for bronchoscopic removal with surgical backup present if needed. Attempts to remove the foreign body in the ED in a stable patient could lead to avoidable and untreatable obstruction. An exception to this rule is the child with epiglottitis. Although progression can be predicted, and airway management difficulty theoretically increases with time, it has been the standard of care to use an expectant approach in children, awaiting definitive airway management if the patient is not in extremis.

Group B represents the group in which expectant treatment of the symptomatic patient is not the best option. This group includes patients with burns, anaphylaxis, caustic ingestions, and trauma. As outlined previously, children are less capable anatomically of accommodating swelling in the airway of any kind, infectious or noninfectious. Those who do not respond to immediate medical treatment if indicated (as in the case of anaphylaxis) should have early intervention to prevent a more difficult, unmanageable problem later.

Other problems, such as the paraairway conditions, need intervention only if symptoms of airway obstruction or failure ensue. The term *paraairway diagnoses* is used to describe conditions involving the airway above the level of the tracheal opening. These conditions rarely require emergency airway intervention of the pediatric patient in the ED.

An example is the retropharyngeal abscess. A retropharyngeal abscess most commonly presents with odynophagia and neck stiffness. Lateral neck films reveal thickening of the retropharyngeal space. Most of these patients have retropharyngeal cellulitis, respond to antibiotics, or if an abscess is truly present, although they require surgical I&D, rarely, if ever, require placement of an airway emergently in the ED. Entities in this category are included in textbooks in the differential of upper-airway obstruction, many times creating the false impression that these are common causes of upper-airway obstruction in children requiring ED intubation. They normally present without the need for emergent airway intervention.

IV. Difficult airways secondary to congenital anomalies

Patients with difficult airways secondary to congenital anomalies receive most attention in discussions of difficult airways in pediatrics. However, they are encountered only rarely in the ED, much less frequently than groups I, II, and III. Also, literature concerning these patients centers on elective situations, managed by experienced pediatric subspecialists, not emergency physicians. Little of the information provided in these discussions is practical therefore for the emergency physician presented with an acute indication for airway management in one of these patients.

Most patients with congenital anomalies presenting to the ED require intubation for reasons that would not be considered difficult in the normal patient. An example is a child with abnormal airway (Pierre-Robin syndrome) who needs mechanical ventilation for respiratory failure secondary to asthma. It is best to be very expectant in the management of these patients, involving pediatric airway specialists at the first sign of impending compromise.

For patients in extremis or crash situations the clinician is left with no other options than those used in other patients. Often such simple procedures as BVM ventilation or endotracheal intubation are successful in these patients and should remain as the mainstay of therapy. Therapeutic options for the pediatric difficult airway are outlined in Table 13.3.

TABLE 13.3. *Therapeutic options*

The difficult airway algorithm applies to children as well as adults with few exceptions; most notably the use of blind nasotracheal intubation is contraindicated below 10 years of age, as is surgical cricothyrotomy. Combitubes, a useful adjunct in adults, are not manufactured for patients with a height of less than 5 feet. Otherwise, the same approach and options are recommended for both children and adults, the only difference being that they are required less often.

There are a variety of airway devices for use in the pediatric patient. However, because of lack of frequency of use except in elective, subspecialty situations, only a few have been used in emergencies and even fewer by emergency physicians. It is probably best to limit the number of options in an effort to gain the maximum experience with them. The following devices and procedures are listed according to appropriateness in different levels of clinical acuity.

Unstable patient
  Noninvasive
    BMV
    BMV + airway
    ET intubation
    Blind NT intubation (>10 yr)
    LMA
  Invasive
    Cricotomes (>5 yr)
    Needle cricothyrotomy
    Surgical cricothyroidotomy (>10 yr)

Semistable Patient
    ET intubation (awake)
    ET intubation (RSI)
    Combitube (>4 ft in height)
    LMA
    Lightwand
    Blind NT intubation (>10 yr)

Stable patient
All emergency departments must have in place a protocol for managing the stable difficult airway foreign body aspiration, epiglottitis, etc. This requires prior agreement of consultants willing to respond immediately to those emergencies.

ADDITIONAL READING

Cote CJ, Todres D. *The pediatric airway in a practice of anesthesia for infants and children,* 2nd ed. Philadelphia: WB Saunders, 1993:55–84.

Raizi, J. The difficult pediatric airway. In: Benumof J, ed. *Airway management: practice and principles.* St Louis: Mosby, 1996:585–637.

Vener P, Lerman J. The pediatric airway and associated syndromes. In: Doyle J, Sandler A, eds. *Anesthesiology clinics of North America.* Philadelphia: WB Saunders, 1995:585–614.

SECTION 3

The Pharmacology
of Airway Management

14

Muscle Relaxants

Robert E. Schneider

Carolinas Medical Center, Department of Emergency Medicine,
Charlotte, North Carolina

I. Neuromuscular blocking agents

Muscle relaxants are the cornerstone of emergency airway management and are used to obtain total control of the patient and to facilitate rapid endotracheal intubation while minimizing the risks of aspiration or other adverse physiologic events. Muscle relaxants do not provide analgesia, sedation, or amnesia, however, and an induction or sedative agent must be used during rapid sequence intubation (RSI) and for post-intubation patient management. There are two classes of muscle relaxants: the noncompetitive or depolarizing neuromuscular blocking agents, of which succinylcholine (Anectine) is the only one in common clinical use, and the two groups of competitive or nondepolarizing agents: the benzylisoquinolinium compounds d-tubocurarine, metocurine, atracurium (Tracrium), cisatracurium (Nimbex), and mivacurium (Mivacron); and the aminosteroid compounds vecuronium (Norcuron), pancuronium (Pavulon), rocuronium (Zemuron), and rapacuronium (Raplon).

II. Noncompetitive depolarizing neuromuscular blocking agent: succinylcholine

The ideal muscle relaxant to facilitate tracheal intubation would have a rapid onset of action, rendering the patient paralyzed within seconds; a short duration of action, returning the patient's normal protective reflexes within 3 to 4 minutes; no significant adverse side effects; and metabolism and excretion independent of liver and kidney function. Unfortunately, such an agent does not exist. Succinylcholine (SCh) comes closest to meeting all these desirable goals. Its drawback, however, is its side effect profile, which will be highlighted later in this section.

SCh is actually two molecules of acetylcholine linked back-to-back and as such, is chemically similar to acetylcholine and stimulates all of the nicotinic and muscarinic cholinergic receptors. Although SCh can be a negative inotrope, this effect is so minimal as to have virtually no clinical relevance. Stimulation of cardiac muscarinic receptors can cause bradycardia, especially in children, but this effect can be blocked by the prior administration of atropine. SCh is a minimal histamine releaser, although this does not appear to have clinical significance. The activity and duration of action of SCh are dependent on rapid hydrolysis by pseudocholinesterase, and ultimately diffusion away from the neuromuscular junction motor endplate, which is devoid of pseudocholinesterase. This is an extremely important pharmacologic concept, as only a fraction of the initial intravenous dose of SCh ever reaches the motor endplate to promote paralysis. It is for this reason that larger, rather than smaller, doses of SCh should always be given in RSI. Incomplete paralysis may jeopardize the patient and may not provide adequate relaxation to facilitate endotracheal intubation. SCh degrades at room temperature, but the degradation is slow and can be mitigated by refrigeration. SCh retains 90% of its activity for up to three months when stored at room temperature. Therefore, SCh can be stored at room temperature for up to three months as long as a quality system is in place to avoid use after this period. One alternative is to place SCh in the ED for one month at room temperature, then exchange it to the OR where it will be refrigerated and rapidly used.

Once SCh reaches the neuromuscular junction, it binds tightly to the acetylcholine receptors, resulting in depolarization that manifests as fasciculations then subsequent paralysis. In the adult patient, the recommended dose of SCh is 1.5mg/kg IV (or 3 mg/kg IM in those very infrequent life-threatening situations wherein IV access is not possible and the airway must be secured immediately). Intravenous administration of SCh results in fasciculations within 10–15 seconds, paralysis within 45–60 seconds, initial return of spontaneous ventilation within 3–5 minutes, and recovery of life sustaining spontaneous ventilation within 8–10 minutes. In children less than 10 years of age, the recommended dose is 2 mg/kg IV, and in the newborn the appropriate dose is 3 mg/kg IV. Because children have higher vagal tone than adults, atropine 0.02 mg/kg IV should be administered as a pretreatment agent to any child under 10 years old who is receiving SCh. Atropine will attenuate the bradycardia produced from both airway manipulation and SCh. This same vagotonic effect must be anticipated in adults when repeated doses of SCh are administered. Succinylmonocholine, the initial metabolite of SCh, sensitizes the cardiac muscarinic receptors in the sinus node to repeat does of SCh. Atropine should be available to reverse bradycardia if it occurs.

It may be impossible in the emergency department to know the exact weight of a patient. In those uncertain circumstances, an additional 20% should be added to the projected dose when calculating the dose of SCh. A 70 kg patient would require 105 mg of SCh (70 kg × 1.5 mg/kg), and to ensure paralysis in cases of dosing uncertainty the administration of 125 mg (20% of 105 = 20 + 105 mg) is recommended. The other option is to administer 2 mg/kg IV to all patients thereby eliminating uncertainty or any miscalculation. There is no harm in giving too much SCh. There are significant downsides to having an inadequately paralyzed patient, i.e., inadequate relaxation, inadequate jaw mobility, and most importantly, the inability to successfully intubate the patient. A straightforward, easy intubation may become a difficult airway, or worse yet, a failed intubation.

A. Side effects of SCh

The recognized side effects of SCh include fasciculations, hyperkalemia, bradycardia, prolonged neuromuscular blockade, malignant hyperthermia, and trismus-masseter muscle spasm. Each of these will be discussed separately.

1. Fasciculations

Fasciculations are thought to be produced by stimulation of the nicotinic acetylcholine receptors. Fasciculation occurs contemporaneously with increases in intracranial pressure, intraocular pressure, intragastric pressure, and has been linked to the muscle pain that can occur following the administration of SCh. The exact mechanisms by which these effects occur are not well elucidated. In patients suspected of having increased intracranial or intraocular pressure, it may be prudent to inhibit these fasciculations. This can be accomplished by giving a defasciculating dose of a nondepolarizing neuromuscular blocking agent such as vecuronium, pancuronium, or rocuronium. Usually 10% of the normal paralyzing dose will be sufficient to inhibit these fasciculations, and recommended doses are 0.01 mg/kg of vecuronium or pancuronium, or 0.1 mg/kg of rocuronium. Administration of any one of these defasciculating agents will abolish the fasciculations and mitigate the rise in intracranial or intraocular pressure. Studies have been variable with respect to prevention of muscle pain, and some patients continue to complain of muscle pain despite the appropriate use of defasciculating agents with SCh, raising further questions regarding the cause and effect. Defasciculating doses of SCh (0.15 mg/kg) given as a pretreatment drug also will inhibit fasciculations but whether this specific pretreatment mitigates any potential rise in intracranial or intraocular pressure is not known. Clinically, inhibition of fasciculations is much more important in the patient with elevated intracranial pressure than in the patient with an open globe injury. The pathophysiologic concern in open globe injury is extrusion of vitreous, which has never been attributed to the administration of SCh. In fact, many anesthesiologists continue to use SCh as a muscle relaxant in cases of open globe injury, with or without an accompanying dose of a defasciculating agent. Similarly, the increase in intragastric pressure that has been measured has never been shown to be of any clinical significance, perhaps because it is offset by a corresponding increase in the distal esophageal sphincter pressure.

2. Hyperkalemia

Under normal circumstances, there may be an increase of up to 0.5 mEq/L of serum potassium associated with normal muscle membrane depolarization following the administration of SCh. In clinical situations of increased receptor density and membrane sensitivity, this increase may approach 5–10 mEq/L and result in hyperkalemic dysrhythmias or cardiac arrest. This results from recruitment and propagation of very sensitive extrajunctional nicotinic receptors that reach action potential following minimal stimuli from depolarizing agents (SCh) and remain depolarized for prolonged periods of time, releasing even larger quantities of potassium. Interestingly, these same extrajunctional nicotinic receptors are relatively refractory to nondepolarizing agents, so that larger doses of vecuronium, pancuronium, or rocuronium will be required to produce paralysis. Fortunately, this hyperkalemia risk does not occur immediately but becomes clinically relevant at varying times (generally 2–7 days post-event), depending on the injury or underlying process. The clinical situations in which this occurs are burns, crush injuries, denervation, and neuromuscular disorders. There have been scattered reports of hyperkalemia following the administration of SCh in patients with severe intraabdominal infections. The clinical relevance of this is not known. Likewise, there is a paucity of evidence supporting the enhancement of hyperkalemia in chronic renal failure patients following the administration of SCh. Indeed, the majority of renal failure patients are successfully intubated using SCh without adverse cardiovascular complications. However, with the advent of newer nondepolarizing agents, there are alternatives to the use of SCh in patients with chronic renal disease, but in the emergency department, SCh remains the drug of choice, except in patients with known hyperkalemia, significant risk of hyperkalemia, or ECG changes suggestive of hyperkalemia. In these situations, rocuronium, vecuronium or rapacuronium would be the muscle relaxants of choice.

In burn victims, the extrajunctional receptor sensitization becomes clinically significant 24 hours post-burn and lasts an indefinite period of time depending on the clinical course of the burn. The percent of body surface area burned does not determine the magnitude of hyperkalemia; significant hyperkalemia has been reported in patients with as little as 10% total body surface area burn, but this is rare. If the burn becomes infected or is delayed in healing, then the patient remains at risk for hyperkalemia throughout the healing phase. It is best not to administer SCh to a burned patient from 24 hours post-burn until 1–2 years following healing of their burned skin. Again, ready availability of rocuronium and rapacuronium for use in burn patients undergoing RSI more than 24 hours post-burn alleviates this concern.

The data regarding crush injuries are scant. The hyperkalemic response begins about 7 days post-injury and persists for 60–90 days, depending on the speed of recovery.

The patient who suffers a denervation event, such as spinal cord injury or stroke, is at risk for hyperkalemia from the end of the first week throughout the first six months following the injury or illness. Patients with neuromuscular disorders such as multiple sclerosis or amyotrophic lateral sclerosis are at risk for hyperkalemia indefinitely, depending on the dynamic state of their disease process. As long as the neuromuscular disease is progressing, there will be augmentation of the extrajunctional receptors and the risk for hyperkalemia. Unlike fasciculations, the hyperkalemic response cannot be attenuated by administering defasciculating doses of nondepolarizing neuromuscular blocking agents, and therefore, these specific clinical situations should be considered absolute contraindications to SCh during the designated time periods.

3. **Bradycardia**

Bradycardia following the administration of SCh is seen most commonly in children due to their heightened vagotonic state. Bradycardia is attenuated or abolished by administering atropine 0.02 mg/kg IV as a pretreatment drug prior to administering SCh. In adults, repeated doses of SCh may produce the same vagotonic effects and administration of atropine may become necessary.

4. **Prolonged neuromuscular blockade**

Prolonged neuromuscular blockade may result from either a congenital absence of pseudocholinesterase or the presence of an atypical form of pseudocholinesterase, either one of which will delay the degradation of SCh and prolong the paralysis. The most common acquired states of pseudocholinesterase deficiency are caused by organophosphate poisoning and cocaine use. Both of these substances poison the enzyme and prolong the effect of SCh. Chronic renal failure, severe liver disease, hypothyroidism, malignancy, malnutrition, pregnancy, cytotoxic drugs, metoclopramide (Reglan) and bambuturol (a long acting beta$_2$-agonist), are but a few of the drugs and clinical conditions that have been implicated as causing acquired deficiencies of pseudocholinesterase and, therefore, prolonging the effects of SCh. Under the very worst of acquired deficiencies, however, the neuromuscular blockade has not been reported to last longer than 20–25 minutes, so SCh is not contraindicated. In the most severe type of congenital pseudocholinesterase deficiency, the blockade can last for several hours.

5. **Malignant hyperthermia**

Malignant hyperthermia (MH) is a genetic skeletal muscle membrane abnormality that can be triggered by halogenated anesthetics, SCh, vigorous exercise, and even emotional stress. Its onset can be acute and progressive or delayed for hours following the initiating event. It is associated with a 60% mortality and is recognized clinically by muscular rigidity, autonomic instability, hypoxia, hypotension, severe lactic acidosis, hyperkalemia, myoglobinemia, and disseminated intravascular coagulation. Elevations in temperature are a late manifestation. Masseter spasm has been claimed to be the hallmark of MH. However, SCh can promote isolated masseter spasm, especially in children, as an exaggerated response at the neuromuscular junction. Therefore, masseter spasm alone is not pathognomonic of MH.

The treatment for MH consists of discontinuing the known or suspected precipitant and the immediate administration of dantrolene sodium (Dantrium). Dantrolene is essential to resuscitation and should be given as soon as the diagnosis is seriously entertained. Dantrolene is a hydantoin derivative that acts directly on skeletal muscle to prevent calcium release from the sarcoplasmic reticulum without affecting calcium reuptake. The initial dose is 2.5 mg/kg IV and is repeated every five minutes until muscle relaxation occurs or the maximum dose of 10 mg/kg is administered. Dantrolene is free of any serious side effects. All cases of MH will require constant monitoring of pH, arterial blood gases, and serum potassium. Immediate and aggressive management of hyperkalemia with the administration of calcium gluconate to antagonize the membrane effects of potassium, or glucose, insulin, and sodium bicarbonate to promote potassium movement intracellularly, may be necessary. A personal or family history of MH is an absolute contraindication to the use of SCh. Interestingly, full paralysis with nondepolarizing neuromuscular blocking agents will prevent SCh-triggered MH. MH has never been reported related to use of SCh in the emergency department. The MH emergency hotline number is (209) 634-4917. Ask for "index zero."

6. **Trismus/masseter muscle spasm**

Whenever SCh is administered, the expected response is paralysis and total relaxation of the patient. On occasion, one may find trismus or masseter muscle spasm following the administration of SCh, especially in children. SCh normally causes a small rise in jaw muscle tension. The normal duration of this response is not known but the spasm is usually transient and should not affect laryngoscopy. Should the trismus or masseter muscle spasm become severe, or progress to involve other muscles of the body then one must consider the development of MH (see above). Pretreatment with nondepolarizing neuromuscular blocking agents will not prevent masseter spasm. If masseter spasm interferes with intubation, a full paralyzing dose of a competitive agent (rocuronium or rapacuronium) should be administered, and the patient should be bag-and-mask ventilated until intubation is possible. In such circumstances, serious consideration should be given to the diagnosis of MH.

B. **Contraindications**

A personal or family history of MH is an absolute contraindication to the use of SCh. Similarly, any patient who is 24 hours or more post-burn, 7 or more days post-crush injury or denervation, or who suffers from a progressive ongoing neuromuscular disease of any etiology should not receive SCh. Relative contraindications to the use of SCh are dependent on the skill and proficiency of the intubator and individual patient circumstances. A patient who is felt to represent a difficult intubation, and in whom ventilation with a bag and mask is also felt to be difficult or impossible, should not receive any neuromuscular blocking agent except as part of a planned approach to the difficult airway. (See Chapters 3 and 5.) In such patients, awake laryngoscopy is strongly recommended before administration of a neuromuscular blocking agent (see Chapters 3 and 7) and preparations should be made for surgical airway access before a neuromuscular blocking agent is administered.

C. **Tips and pearls**

• SCh 1.5 mg/kg IV or 3 mg/kg IM in the adult, 2 mg/kg IV in the child less than 10 years old, and 3 mg/kg IV in the infant or neonate remains the muscle relaxant of choice for RSI in the emergency department. This is due to its rapid production of paralysis (45–60 seconds), and its relatively short duration of action (6–10 minutes).

- The side effect profile of SCh should prompt careful deliberation under specific clinical situations, but in most circumstances, SCh can be administered safely and effectively. In the National Emergency Airway Registry (NEAR) pilot study of almost 6000 intubations in 24 centers, SCh was used safely and successfully for the vast majority of intubations.
- Pretreating patients prior to the administration of SCh with a defasciculating dose of a nondepolarizing neuromuscular blocking agent is probably only required when the patient has known or suspected elevated intracranial pressure. If hyperkalemia is suspected, a competitive (nondepolarizing) agent should be used in place of SCh.
- SCh should be avoided in burn patients (after 24 hours), crush injury patients (after 7 days), patients with active intraabdominal infections (after 7 days), and those patients suffering denervation (after 7 days) or neuromuscular disease (after 7 days).
- SCh is contraindicated in patients with a personal or family history of MH.

III. Competitive, nondepolarizing neuromuscular blocking agents

The competitive, nondepolarizing neuromuscular blocking agents actually compete with and block the action of acetylcholine at the neuromuscular junction receptor site, thereby causing paralysis. Because there is competitive blockade, rather than stimulation of the receptor site, there are no fasciculations. The competitive, nondepolarizing neuromuscular blocking agents of clinical significance are divided into two groups: the benzylisoquinolinum compounds (atracurium and mivacurium) and the aminosteroid compounds (vecuronium, pancuronium, rocuronium and rapacuronium). Of the two groups, the aminosteroid compounds are the only agents used commonly in the emergency department for RSI. Their primary use is in cases where SCh is contraindicated, for all cases of initial post-intubation patient management and as a defasciculating agent in patients with elevated ICP. On occasion the defasciculating dose will render the patient weak or even totally paralyzed and apneic. Therefore, one must always be prepared to accelerate the RSI algorithms and rapidly administer the remainder of the paralyzing dose of muscle relaxant and intubate the trachea.

Of the four aminosteroid compounds, pancuronium is the least expensive but may be less desirable because it has a tendency to produce tachycardia by competitive cardiac muscarinic blockade. Vecuronium and rocuronium are more expensive but do not promote tachycardia. All of the competitive nondepolarizing neuromuscular blocking agents are generally less desirable for intubation than SCh because of either delayed time to paralysis, prolonged duration of action, or both. Their time to paralysis can be shortened by increasing the paralyzing dose but this further prolongs the duration of action. This can complicate management of failed airway situations if the patient cannot be successfully intubated or oxygenated. Even with SCh, complete recovery of life sustaining spontaneous ventilation cannot be expected until well after critical hemoglobin desaturation has occurred. Rocuronium and most recently, rapacuronium, are the only aminosteroid compounds whose time to onset of paralysis closely parallels that of SCh.

Rapacuronium, an analogue of vecuronium, is the latest in a series of new aminosteroid compounds whose accelerated time to onset is attributable to its low potency. Although its onset is rapid, some studies have questioned its variability on intrinsic laryngeal muscle relaxation at paralyzing doses of 1.5 mg/kg. However, most clinical studies have identified good to excellent intubating conditions with 1.5 mg/kg of RAP within 60 seconds of administration. Rapacuronium's side effect profile is somewhat concerning as tachycardia, transient hypotension, and clinically significant bronchospasm have been reported in studies comparing rapacuronium to SCh. This is in contrast with the very favorable side effect profiles of the other aminosteroids and requires further study. The use of competitive agents for RSI is discussed in detail in Chapter 7. Table 14-1 lists the onset and duration of action of all the neuromuscular blocking drugs.

A unique feature of all the competitive nondepolarizing neuromuscular blocking agents is that they can be reversed by administering acetylcholinesterase inhibitors such as neostigmine (Prostigmine) 0.06–0.08 mg/kg IV. These enzyme inhibitors will not become clinically effective in longer acting muscle relaxants (pancuronium, vecuronium, rocuronium) until significant (40%) spontaneous recovery has occurred. At this point, the prevention of acetylcholine metabolism by the inhibitors will allow increasing concentrations of acetylcholine to bathe the neuromuscular junction where it will selectively bind onto two alpha subunits of the protein receptor and promote full neuromuscular recovery. Atropine 0.02 mg/kg IV or glycopyrrolate (Robinul) 0.2 mg IV should be available to counteract any excessive muscarinic stimulation. Due to the required percent of spontaneous recovery that is needed before clinically apparent reversal is appreciated, these inhibitory agents are rarely recommended for emergency department use following the administration of pancuronium, vecuronium, or rocuronium, and should not be depended on in cases of failed tracheal intubation. One of the most attractive benefits of rapacuronium, however, in addition to its rapid onset, is its accelerated reversal by neostigmine without required time for spontaneous recovery. This effect is most likely attributable to its low potency. Neostigmine will reduce the recovery time from 1.5 mg/kg of rapacuronium to 11 minutes (similar to SCh) from 24 minutes. This scenario will require access to and proficiency with another drug (neostigmine), but may result in an acceptable alternative in patients in whom SCh is contraindicated. Subsequent studies will define the optimum role of rapacuronium in RSI.

A. Tips and pearls

- The use of nondepolarizers during the pretreatment phase in those patients at risk for increases in intracranial pressure requires 10% of the normal paralyzing dose. Although uncommon, this reduced dose may render the patient weak or totally paralyzed, in which case acceleration of the RSI algorithm will be required.

TABLE 14-1. *Onset and duration of action of neuromuscular blocking drugs*

Drug	Dose (mg/kg)	Time to maximal blockade	Time to recovery (min) 25%	Time to recovery (min) 75%
Quarternary amine				
Succinylcholine	1.0	1.1	8	11 (90%)
Benzylisoquinolinium compounds				
Tubocurarine	0.5	3.4	—	130
Metocurine	0.4	4.1	107	—
Alcuronium	0.2	7.1	47 (20%)	90 (70%)
Atracurium	0.4	2.4	38	52
Doxacurium	0.05	5.9	83	116
Mivacurium	0.15	1.8	16	25
Cisatracirium	0.1	7.7	46	63
Aminosteroid compounds				
Pancuronium	0.08	2.9	86	—
Vecoronium	0.1	2.4	44	56
Pipecuronium	0.07	2.5	95	136
Rocuronium	0.6	1.0	43	66
Rapacuronium[a]	1.5	1.4	10.7	24 (70%)

Hunter JM. Drug therapy: new neuromuscular blocking drugs. *N Engl J Med* 1995;332:1691–1699.
[a] Goulden MR, Hunter JM. Editorial I Rapacuronium (org. 9487): do we have a replacement for succinylcholine? *Br J Anaesthesia* 1999;82:489–492.

- The principal use of competitive nondepolarizing neuromuscular blocking agents is during the initial phase of post-intubation patient management.
- Nondepolarizers are also used as the primary muscle relaxant in those patients who either have contraindications to the use of SCh or when the physician prefers the drug for personal reasons. If vecuronium is used, even in the increased dose of 0.3 mg/kg, one must be prepared for a longer time to onset of paralysis (90 seconds). With 1.0 mg/kg of rocuronium, or 1.5 mg/kg of rapacuronium, intubating level paralysis will occur in a time comparable to that of SCh, 45–60 seconds. In any case, when a nondepolarizing agent is used, duration of action is much longer (VEC: 110 minutes, ROC: 40 minutes, RAP: 23 minutes).
- Rapacuronium may prove to be a suitable substitute for SCh in RSI if subsequent studies confirm its clinical efficacy regarding accelerated time to recovery and its side effect profile compares favorably with other aminosteroids.

ADDITIONAL READING

Bishop MJ, Bedford RF, Kil HK. Physiologic and pathophysiologic responses to intubation. In: Benumof JL, ed. *Airway management principles and practice*. St Louis: Mosby, 1996:102–117.

Lev R, Rosen P. Prophylactic lidocaine use preintubation: a review. *J Emerg Med* 1994;12:4;499–506.

Miller RD. Pharmacology of muscle relaxants and their antagonists. In: Miller RD, ed. *Anesthesia*, 4th ed. New York: Churchill Livingstone, 1994:417–487.

Schmutz DW, Muhlebach SF. Stability of succinylcholine chloride injection. *Am J Health Syst Pharm* 1991;48:501.

15

Sedatives and Induction Agents

Robert E. Schneider

*Carolinas Medical Center, Department of Emergency Medicine,
Charlotte, North Carolina*

The ideal induction agent would smoothly and quickly render the patient unconscious, unresponsive, and amnestic in one arm/heart/brain circulation time. Such an agent would also provide analgesia, maintain stable cerebral perfusion pressure and cardiovascular hemodynamics, be immediately reversible, and have few, if any, adverse side effects. Unfortunately, such an induction agent does not exist. Most induction agents do meet the first criteria because they are highly lipophilic and therefore have a rapid onset within 15 to 30 seconds of intravenous administration. Their clinical effect is likewise terminated quickly as the drug rapidly redistributes to less-well-perfused tissues. All the induction agents have the potential to cause myocardial depression and subsequent hypotension. These effects depend on the particular drug, the patient's underlying physiologic condition, and the dose and speed of injection of the drug. The faster the drug is administered (intravenous [IV] push), the larger the concentration of drug that saturates those organs with the greatest blood flow (i.e., brain and heart) and the more pronounced the effect. Because rapid sequence intubation (RSI) requires rapid administration of the sedative/induction agent, the choice of drug and the dose must be individualized.

The induction agents are classified as sedatives/hypnotics and include ultra-short-acting barbiturates: thiopental (Pentothal) and methohexital (Brevital); benzodiazepines: midazolam (Versed); and miscellaneous agents: etomidate (Amidate), ketamine (Ketalar), and propofol (Diprivan).

I. Ultra-short-acting barbiturates
A. Thiopental (Pentothal)
Thiopental is the prototypical barbiturate. These agents act at the barbiturate receptor, which forms part of the GABA-receptor complex to enhance and mimic the action of GABA. Thiopental decreases GABA dissociation from its receptor, which enhances GABA's neuroinhibitory activity, directly opens the chloride channel, and—at higher drug concentrations—causes hyperpolarization of this chloride channel.

Thiopental is cerebroprotective and its primary use is as an induction agent. Thiopental may be used in the emergency department (ED) for patients who are suspected of having increased intracranial pressure and require tracheal intubation. Thiopental causes a dose-dependent decrease in cerebral metabolic oxygen consumption and a parallel decrease in cerebral blood flow and intracranial pressure, while maintaining cerebral perfusion pressure in a steady state. Thiopental has long been one of the most commonly used sedative hypnotic agents for RSI and for rapid sequence induction of anesthesia. Its rapid onset, brief duration, and relatively predictable side effect profile make it an excellent induction agent.

The dosing of thiopental depends on the hemodynamic status of the patient and the concomitant use of other agents in the RSI algorithm. Thiopental is a potent venodilator and myocardial depressant. Consequently, the dose must be decreased in the elderly and whenever it is used with other drugs that affect the sympathetic, cardiac, or respiratory systems. In euvolemic adults, the recommended induction dose is 3 to 5 mg/kg IV. In the euvolemic child and infant, the dose is 5 to 8 mg/kg IV. In the hypovolemic patient or patient in whom the volume status is unknown, the adult dose is 1 to 3 mg/kg IV and the pediatric dose is 1 to 5 mg/kg IV. The time to onset is 15 to 30 seconds with full recovery because of drug redistribution in 3 to 5 minutes. Thiopental should be avoided entirely in profoundly hypotensive patients for whom other drugs, especially etomidate and ketamine, may preserve greater hemodynamic stability.

The chief side effects of thiopental include central respiratory depression, venodilation, and myocardial depression. These latter two may be manifested by hypotension that tends to be greater in both treated and untreated hypertensive patients compared with normotensive patients. Thiopental causes a dose-related release of histamine that in most situations is not clinically significant. As with any induction agent, inadequate dosing leaves the patient more lightly sedated and susceptible to laryngospasm from any pharyngolaryngeal stimulation prior to the administration and onset of a muscle relaxant. Despite the fact that thiopental crosses the placenta, there is reported fetal safety to 6 mg/kg IV. Larger doses may produce fetal cardiovascular depression. One to two percent of patients will experience pain on injection of thiopental, especially if small veins on the dorsum of the hand are utilized. Inadvertent intraarterial injection or subcutaneous extravasation of thiopental can result in chemical endarteritis and distal thrombosis, ischemia, and tissue necrosis. Should extravasation occur, 40 to 80 mg of papaverine (Cerespan) in 20 ml normal saline or 10 ml of 1% lidocaine (Xylocaine) should be injected intraarterially proximal to the site. Thiopental is absolutely contraindicated in those patients with acute intermittent porphyria, or variegate porphyria, as it can activate the enzyme responsible for precipitating an acute attack.

B. Methohexital (Brevital)

Methohexital shares similar pharmacologic properties with thiopental. It is two to three times more potent than thiopental, 1.5 mg of methohexital being equal to 4 mg of thiopental. The time to onset is faster and the duration of action shorter with methohexital. As a rule, the more rapid the onset of a drug, the more profound the adverse effects (e.g., hypotension, respiratory depression). In the euvolemic patient, 1.5 mg/kg IV is the recommended dose. In the hypovolemic or unknown volume status patient, 0.5 mg/kg IV should be administered. Methohexital causes more excitatory phenomena (twitching, hiccups) than thiopental. In about 5% of patients there is pain on drug injection, and as with thiopental, methohexital crosses the placenta. Methohexital is often used in those patients undergoing cardioversion or electroconvulsive therapy where rapid onset of amnesia and a short duration of action are the primary pharmacotherapeutic effects being recruited. As an agent for RSI, thiopental is probably preferable to methohexital, but both have been widely and successfully used.

1. Tips and pearls

For years thiopental has been the standard induction agent of choice for RSI. However, with the development of newer, more versatile agents with fewer significant side effects, its use has diminished. Its side effect profile—namely, venodilation and myocardial depression—can be detrimental in many patients in whom optimal preload is required to maintain cardiac output and prevent organ ischemia. In terms of drug preparation and administration, both thiopental and methohexital are not user-friendly. Both drugs come in a powder form that requires reconstitution that at times makes emergency administration awkward. Thiopental may be particularly desirable in patients undergoing RSI for status epilepticus, as it shares anticonvulsant properties with the other sedative hypnotics.

II. Benzodiazepines

Similar to the barbiturates, the benzodiazepines work at the GABA-receptor complex. Benzodiazepines specifically stimulate the benzodiazepine receptor, which in turn modulates GABA, the primary neuroinhibitory transmitter. The benzodiazepines provide amnesia, anxiolysis, central muscle relaxation, sedation, anticonvulsant effects, and hypnosis. Their direct effect on intracranial pressure is controversial. The amnestic properties of the benzodiazepines are their greatest asset and are dose related. The lipophilicity of the benzodiazepines varies widely. The more lipid soluble the benzodiazepine, the quicker time to onset and offset. Midazolam (Versed) is the most lipid soluble of the benzodiazepines and therefore has a more rapid onset (30 to 60 seconds) than diazepam (Valium) (45 to 90 seconds), which in turn has a more rapid onset than lorazepam (Ativan) (60 to 120 seconds). Regardless, the time to onset of benzodiazepines is longer than that of the barbiturates. The termination of action of these drugs is due to redistribution and then metabolism via hepatic microsomal oxidation for midazolam and diazepam and glucuronide conjugation for lorazepam. Diazepam has two active metabolites, the clinical significance of which is unknown. Midazolam has one slightly active metabolite and lorazepam has five inactive metabolites. As expected, the pharmacokinetic variables for the three benzodiazepines are quite different, with the half-life for midazolam being 1.7 to 2.6 hours; that for lorazepam, 11 to 22 hours; and that for diazepam, 20 to 50 hours. The benzodiazepines, in general, are free of allergic reactions.

The primary indications for benzodiazepines are to promote amnesia and sedation. In this regard, the benzodiazepines are unparalleled. Unfortunately, there is great variability in dosing requirements among patients. Men seem to be more sensitive to the drug than women, and the elderly are more sensitive than younger patients. Therefore appropriate dosing can be challenging. The standard induction dose of midazolam is 0.2 mg/kg IV; of diazepam, 0.3 to 0.5 mg/kg IV; and of lorazepam, 0.1 mg/kg IV. There is a dose-related reduction in systemic vascular resistance and direct myocardial depression at induction doses of midazolam. Very rarely is a full induction dose of any benzodiazepine administered because of their dosing variability, fears (perhaps unfounded) of potentially harmful side effects, and lack of familiarity of physicians with the appropriate induction doses. Physicians tend to use benzodiazepines for procedural sedation, which requires a lower dose, and may not be aware of proper induction doses. The benzodiazepines, like the barbiturates, cross the placenta but cause less fetal depression at equipotent doses than do the barbiturates.

1. Tips and pearls

The benzodiazepines provide unparalleled amnesia. However, their slower onset, greater dosing variability among patients of all ages, and side effect profile (i.e., myocardial depression and hypotension) make them relatively less attractive than etomidate as induction agents for RSI in the ED. However, the amnestic properties of the benzodiazepines are unsurpassed and occur even at suboptimal induction doses. Midazolam therefore remains an option and an important adjunct for RSI. Benzodiazepines are effective and safe for maintenance of sedation after intubation is achieved (e.g., diazepam 0.2 mg/kg initially, then approximately 20% to 30% of this dose repeated every 30 to 60 minutes as needed).

III. Miscellaneous agents

A. Etomidate (Amidate)

Etomidate is an imidazole derivative that is primarily a hypnotic. It is the most hemodynamically stable of the currently available induction agents. At induction doses of 0.2 to 0.3 mg/kg IV, it causes minimal respiratory or myocardial depression. Etomidate attenuates both underlying elevated intracranial pressure and further increases that are associated with laryngoscopy and intubation. It does this by decreasing cerebral blood flow and cerebral metabolic oxygen demand without adversely affecting cerebral perfusion pressure (Chapter 19). In healthy, hemodynamically stable patients, the recommended induction dose of 0.3 mg/kg should be used. The onset is 20 to 30 seconds, with full recovery in 7 to 14 minutes.

Etomidate does not release histamine, but it can cause nausea and vomiting, pain on injection, myoclonic movement, and hiccups. The 30% to 40% incidence of nausea and vomiting on emergence from etomidate induction compares with a 10% to 20% incidence following administration of thiopental or methohexital. This is not usually an issue in the ED, where patients are usually kept sedated and paralyzed after tracheal intubation. A small number of patients will experience pain on injection of etomidate. This is due to the diluent (propylene glycol) and can be lessened considerably if administered in a large vein (e.g., an antecubital vein) in conjunction with a rapid intravenous fluid rate. The myoclonic activity following etomidate injection is caused by brain stem stimulation and might be mistaken for seizure activity. This myoclonus can be mitigated, if desired, by the concomitant administration of small doses of benzodiazepines or opioids, but this is generally not necessary for RSI in the ED because neuromuscular blocking agents are being given. Hiccups are usually not a concern during RSI but should be recognized as a side effect of etomidate administration.

The best-known and most disconcerting side effect of etomidate is its reversible blockade of 11-beta-hydroxylase, which decreases both serum cortisol and aldosterone levels. This side effect has been more common with continuous infusions of etomidate in the intensive care unit setting than with a single-dose injection utilized for RSI. Adverse effects due to cortisol suppression have not been reported in ED patients undergoing RSI.

1. Tips and pearls

Etomidate has become a very popular induction agent because of its cerebroprotective effect and its unique hemodynamic stability. Etomidate maintains cerebral perfusion pressure in most clinical situations. As with any induction agent, the dose should be reduced in cases of hypotension or decreased intravascular volume, but etomidate exhibits the best balance of utility and safety of all the induction agents under consideration. In more unstable patients, 0.15 mg/kg IV of etomidate coupled with 1.5 mg/kg IV succinylcholine in a rapid sequence technique will produce excellent intubating conditions quickly, maintain cerebral and myocardial perfusion, and return the patient to an awake state in 7 to 14 minutes. In healthy, euvolemic patients, 0.3 mg/kg IV should be used. Cortisol suppression is not a concern in the ED.

B. Ketamine (Ketalar)

Ketamine is a PCP derivative that provides excellent analgesia, anesthesia, and amnesia. The amnestic effect, however, is not as pronounced as that seen with the benzodiazepines. Ketamine releases catecholamines and therefore augments heart rate and blood pressure in those patients who are not already maximally sympathetically stimulated. It increases cerebral cortical activity and may potentiate increases in intracranial pressure. Therefore, despite recent studies that have challenged this concept, ketamine should be considered to be relatively contraindicated in those patients with known or suspected increased intracranial pressure. In addition to its catecholamine-releasing effect, ketamine directly relaxes bronchial smooth muscle, producing bronchodilation. It is the induction agent of choice for bronchospastic patients who require tracheal intubation. Because of its pharmacologic profile, ketamine also should be considered the induction agent of choice for patients who are hypovolemic or hypotensive without evidence of serious head injury and for patients with hemodynamic instability due to cardiac tamponade or intrinsic myocardial disease but without ischemic heart disease. In patients with ischemic heart disease, catecholamine release may adversely increase myocardial oxygen demand. The induction dose of ketamine is 1 to 2 mg/kg IV. The onset of action is 15 to 30 seconds, the duration is 10 to 15 minutes, and full recovery occurs in 15 to 30 minutes. In doses greater than 1.5 mg/kg IV, ketamine may cause myocardial depression. Because of its stimulating effects, ketamine enhances laryngeal reflexes, increases pharyngeal and bronchial secretions, and may precipitate laryngospasm. Atropine 0.02 mg/kg IV or glycopyrrolate (Robinul) 0.005 mg/kg IV may be administered in conjunction with ketamine to promote a drying effect. The hallucinations that are well known to occur occasionally on emergence from ketamine are more common in the adult than in the child and can be eliminated by the concomitant or subsequent administration of a benzodiazepine, if desired. This is rarely an issue in ED airway management, in which the patient is usually sedated for prolonged periods, often with benzodiazepines.

1. Tips and pearls

Ketamine is the induction agent of choice in asthmatics or other patients with reactive airways disease who require tracheal intubation. It should also be considered the induction agent of choice in patients who are hypotensive or hypovolemic without evidence of acute severe brain injury. Even in hypotensive patients with acute brain injury, ketamine may be an acceptable choice. Cerebral perfusion pressure equals mean arterial pressure minus intracranial pressure, and maintenance of mean arterial pressure may circumvent any rise in intracranial pressure if other agents are available. However, ketamine is generally avoided in patients with suspected increased intracranial pressure if other agents are available (Chapter 19). In unusual circumstances, if ketamine must be given intramuscularly, the induction dose is 4 to 6 mg/kg IM.

C. **Propofol (Diprivan)**

Propofol is an alkylphenol derivative with hypnotic properties. It is highly lipid soluble. At typical induction doses, it attenuates potential rises in intracranial pressure but does so at the expense of cerebral perfusion pressure. It is also a myocardial depressant. For these reasons it is rarely, if ever, the induction agent of choice in the ED. Propofol has pharmacologic properties similar to both thiopental and etomidate. It causes greater myocardial depression and venodilation than thiopental. It produces excellent sedation and causes minimal, if any, cortisol suppression compared with etomidate. There have been reports in the literature of propofol's use as an induction agent during tracheal intubation for reactive airways disease. The pharmacotherapeutics in this specific clinical scenario seem to parallel those of ketamine. The induction dose of propofol is 0.5 to 1.2 mg/kg IV.

1. Tips and pearls

Propofol has little utility as an induction agent in the ED because of its side effect profile, which consists mainly of hypotension and reduction in cerebral perfusion pressure and general lack of familiarity with this drug in the ED. Most often selection of one of the other induction agents will be more appropriate.

ADDITIONAL READING

Ko S, Kim DC, Han YJ, Song HS. Small dose fentanyl: optimal time of injection for blunting the circulatory responses to tracheal intubation. *Anesth Analg* 1998;86:658–661.

Miller RD. Barbiturates. In: Miller RD, ed. *Anesthesia,* 4th ed. New York: Churchill Livingstone, 1994:229–246.

Miller RD. Nonbarbiturate intravenous anesthetics. In: Miller RD, ed. *Anesthesia,* 4th ed. New York: Churchill Livingstone, 1994:247–289.

16

Drugs for Special Clinical Circumstances

Robert E. Schneider

Carolinas Medical Center, Department of Emergency Medicine,
Charlotte, North Carolina

I. Neuroleptics

Neuroleptic agents are often used in the emergency department (ED) for their potent central calming effect with minimal respiratory or hemodynamic consequences. When a combative patient presents to the ED, it is important to identify the etiology of the combativeness so that subsequent decisions can be made that will be most beneficial to the patient's outcome. It must be determined whether the combativeness is metabolic, structural, or simply a manifestation of drug or alcohol intoxication. The decision process between neurolepsis and rapid sequence intubation (RSI) is described in Chapter 18.

There are two main classes of neuroleptics: phenothiazines and butyrophenones. Phenothiazines tend to promote hypotension and are therefore less appropriate for patient control in the ED. The butyrophenones, haloperidol (Haldol) and droperidol (Inapsine), are lipophilic amines that bind to the GABA receptors on the postsynaptic membrane as well as the reuptake sites for dopamine, norepinephrine, acetylcholine, histamine, and serotonin. The binding affinity of these drugs determines their pharmacologic effect as well as their side effect profile. Both drugs have minimal potential to affect respiratory drive or hemodynamics adversely and are the agents of choice for control of combative behavior in the ED.

Haloperidol is administered intravenously in 5- to 10-mg increments every 3 to 10 minutes until the desired effect is achieved. Droperidol has a quicker onset and offset, is less likely to produce dystonic reactions, and is a more potent sedative and antiemetic than haloperidol. Droperidol is administered intravenously 2.5 to 5 mg every 5 minutes until the desired effect is achieved.

Alpha-adrenergic receptor blockade tends to be more common and more pronounced with droperidol than with haloperidol. Hypotension may occur in the hypovolemic patient, or the patient dependent on sympathetic stimulation to maintain blood pressure. However, this effect is usually self-limited or responsive to intravenous (IV) fluids. Neuroleptic malignant syndrome is a rare but serious side effect of neuroleptic agents. This is a central disorder of thermoregulation that is usually seen at drug initiation or with any increase in drug dosing. These patients experience muscular rigidity that does not respond to the usual antagonists, may manifest temperatures to 107 degrees, and suffer from altered mental status and autonomic instability. The treatment of neuroleptic malignant syndrome consists of cessation of the responsible drug, administration of dantrolene (Dantrium) similar to malignant hyperthermia (Chapter 14), and the use of benzodiazepines as needed for sedation and anxiolysis. The neuromuscular junction is unaffected by neuroleptic malignant syndrome and will be normally responsive to muscle relaxants if required to reverse muscle rigidity or perform tracheal intubation.

A. Tips and pearls

The neuroleptic agents can be tremendously helpful in controlling acute psychosis or drug- or alcohol-induced inappropriate patient behavior in the ED. In those situations unrelated to drugs or alcohol, recognition and correction of the underlying pathophysiologic process (hypoxia, hypoglycemia) may help to control the patient's behavior. The safety profile of the neuroleptic agents makes them attractive for use in the ED. In particular, both haloperidol and droperidol possess extremely safe respiratory and hemodynamic profiles.

II. Drugs used in the pretreatment phase of RSI

A. General approach

During the pretreatment phase of RSI, a decision must be made about administration of specific drugs that will attenuate the normal physiologic and pathophysiologic reflex responses caused by airway manipulation (laryngoscopy) and the insertion of an endotracheal tube (intubation). These reflex responses are initiated by stimulation of afferent receptors in the posterior pharynx, hypopharynx, and larynx, which result in increased afferent traffic and central stimulation of the brain leading to increases in intracranial pressure (ICP), stimulation of the autonomic nervous system leading to increases in heart rate and blood pressure, and stimulation of the upper and lower respiratory tract resulting in increases in airway resistance. It is well known that the duration (>15 seconds) and aggressiveness of laryngoscopy and stimulation of the carina are factors that initiate and augment these reflex responses. The central nervous system, cardiovascular system, and respiratory system all respond predictably to these stimuli, and in selected patients, the resultant physiologic manifestations may adversely affect the patient's outcome. Even though well-controlled outcome studies have not been done, it seems reasonable, given the available data, that all attempts should be made to attenuate these responses and to use pharmacologic agents that mitigate the patient's underlying or presenting problems.

The central nervous system responds to airway manipulation by increasing cerebral metabolic oxygen demand, increasing cerebral blood flow, and, if intracranial elastance is compromised, increasing ICP. This is important in situations in which there is loss of autoregulation such that blood flow to the brain or regions of the brain is pressure passive (i.e., increases in blood pressure result in increases in ICP).

The cardiovascular system responds to the sympathetic nervous system actuation triggered by airway stimulation. In children this is seen primarily as a monosynaptic reflex promoting vagal stimulation of the SA node that results in bradycardia. In adults, a polysynaptic event predominates, whereby impulses travel afferently via the 9th and 10th cranial nerves to the brain stem and spinal cord, and then return efferently through the cardioaccelerator nerves and sympathetic ganglia. This results in norepinephrine release from the adrenergic nerve terminals, epinephrine release from the adrenal glands, and activation of the renin-angiotensin system, which further leads to increases in blood pressure. This overall increase in heart rate and blood pressure to levels as high as twice normal may be detrimental in those patients with myocardial ischemia, with known aortic or intracerebral aneurysm or dissection, or with a penetrating trauma where any increase in shear pressure may reactivate previous hemorrhage.

The respiratory system responds in two important ways to airway stimulation. There is activation of the upper-airway reflexes that can lead to laryngospasm and coughing, both of which compromise the patient. Of these, the former is obviously more significant in producing a difficult airway situation. However, neuromuscular blockade abolishes laryngospasm. Coughing may be significant in cases of increased ICP, fractured vertebrae, or penetrating globe injuries. In all patients, there is actuation of the lower-airway reflexes that leads to increases in airway resistance. This is most often manifested by bronchospasm, which can be reflex, irritant, or antigenic in nature and can result in significant morbidity.

Whether control of these adverse reflexes improves patient outcome is not yet known, but the body of knowledge that is currently available argues for the use of specific pretreatment drugs capable of mitigating potentially harmful physiologic effects. To optimize their effect, all these pretreatment agents should be administered 3 minutes before induction, if possible. The goal is to achieve peak drug concentration at the precise time the patient is undergoing laryngoscopy and intubation. The uses of the individual drugs in specific clinical circumstances are described in Chapters 16 to 24. The useful agents are most easily remembered by the mnemonic *LOAD,* which stands for *L*idocaine, *O*pioid, *A*tropine, and *D*efasciculating agent. This chapter provides a general discussion of the appropriate pharmacologic agents and their relevant properties.

B. The LOAD approach

1. Lidocaine (Xylocaine)

The literature is replete with articles that debate the efficacy of lidocaine in the pretreatment phase of tracheal intubation. It has been shown unequivocally that 1.5 mg/kg of lidocaine IV 3 minutes before intubation suppresses the cough reflex and attenuates the increase in airway resistance that is irritant in origin (endotracheal tube). Its effect on antigenic bronchospasm is more controversial. The literature is likewise supportive of lidocaine's mitigating effect on potential increases in ICP at 1.5 mg/kg IV 3 minutes before tracheal intubation. This is ascribed to lidocaine's ability to increase the depth of anesthesia, decrease cerebral metabolic oxygen demand globally, decrease cerebral blood flow, and increase cerebrovascular resistance. The literature is indecisive and indeed contradictory regarding lidocaine's effect on attenuating the sympathetic response to laryngoscopy, and therefore lidocaine cannot be recommended for this purpose.

a. Tips and pearls

The use of 1.5 mg/kg IV lidocaine 3 minutes before induction is advocated for all patients with reactive airway disease (tight lungs) or elevated ICP (tight brains) (Chapters 19 and 20). Lidocaine has a wide safety profile at 1.5 mg/kg IV. The primary toxic effect is the development of seizures, which should only occur at much greater doses. The effect of 4% topical lidocaine on ICP or airway reactivity is incompletely studied and this agent should be reserved for use during awake intubation techniques (Chapter 8).

2. Opioid—fentanyl (Sublimaze)

Given in sufficiently high doses, most anesthetic agents, with the exception of ketamine, will attenuate the reflex sympathetic response to laryngoscopy. However, the doses and depth of anesthesia that are required to achieve substantial attenuation will produce significant hypotension. The opioids, specifically fentanyl, significantly attenuate this sympathetic response with minimal side effects. Fentanyl has no direct effect on ICP. However, increasing doses of any of the opioids will suppress ventilation, resulting in hypercarbia, cerebrovasodilation, and subsequent increases in ICP. Fentanyl does not release histamine and has no direct effect on the pulmonary response to laryngoscopy. Fentanyl has been shown to have a partial attenuating effect on the reflex sympathetic response to laryngoscopy at doses as low as 2 µg/kg IV.

A greater response with moderate attenuation is seen at 6 µg/kg IV, and almost complete attenuation at 11 to 15 µg/kg IV, a rather large dose and one usually reserved for patients undergoing cardiac surgery.

In the ED, a dose of 3 µg/kg of fentanyl IV 3 minutes before intubation is indicated for patients who might be adversely affected by any transient increase in heart rate or blood pressure (Chapters 19 and 22). Patients with elevated ICP, ischemic heart disease, known or suspected cerebral or aortic aneurysm, aortic dissection, and perhaps hemodynamically stable penetrating trauma are all candidates for pretreatment with fentanyl.

Fentanyl should be given as the last of the pretreatment drugs, over an interval of 30 to 60 seconds. Caution must be used when fentanyl is given as a pretreatment agent because significant respiratory depression and hypotension (central sympathectomy) may occur. Muscle wall rigidity is a unique and idiosyncratic response to opioids and is probably related to the dose and speed of opioid administration, the concomitant use of nitrous oxide, and the presence or absence of muscle relaxants. It is not reversible with naloxone (Narcan). It is usually seen with fentanyl doses well in excess of 500 µg and primarily affects the chest and abdominal wall musculature. The rigidity is infrequently seen in conscious patients and tends to occur very quickly after the patient begins to lose consciousness. Rigidity has not been reported with the ED use of fentanyl. Rigidity can be attenuated or prevented with defasciculating doses of a nondepolarizing neuromuscular blocking agent or by the administration of paralyzing doses of succinylcholine (SCh) once the abnormality is recognized. Avoiding the rapid administration of large doses of opioids is the most reliable way of avoiding this complication. Fentanyl dosing must be tailored when used in conjunction with other induction agents.

a. Tips and pearls

In the operating room, fentanyl is used as an induction agent at doses of 15 to 30 µg/kg IV. In the ED, fentanyl is a pretreatment agent, not an induction agent. Fentanyl has its greatest utility in those patients at risk from increasing blood pressure (i.e., increases in ICP, myocardial pressure [ischemia], or vascular shear pressure [aneurysmal disease, dissection, penetrating vascular trauma]). In these patients any further increase in sympathetic stimulation from laryngoscopy and intubation might be detrimental to the patient's outcome. One must be prepared for dose-related hypotension and respiratory depression that may occur with fentanyl administration.

3. Atropine

Atropine is indicated in only two clinical situations in the ED. All children less than 10 years of age should be pretreated with atropine 0.02 mg/kg IV 3 minutes before the administration of SCh. Any adult who receives a second dose of SCh is at risk for augmentation of vagal tone and atropine 0.5 to 2 mg IV should be available to counteract this vagotonic effect.

4. Defasciculating Agents

Defasciculating agents applicable to the pretreatment phase of RSI include the aminosteroid nondepolarizing muscle relaxants vecuronium, pancuronium, and rocuronium. Their greatest utility is mitigating potential increases in ICP caused by SCh; therefore they should be considered for use in all medical and trauma situations in which increases in ICP are a concern and SCh is selected as the muscle relaxant (Chapter 19). These drugs do not attenuate the reflex sympathetic response to laryngoscopy, nor do they attenuate increases in airway resistance. The appropriate defasciculating dose for any of these agents is 10% of the normal paralyzing dose.

With any of the nondepolarizing neuromuscular blocking agents, the defasciculating dose may uncommonly cause muscular weakness or even apnea. Tracheal intubation may need to be completed quickly should this occur. Pancuronium can cause tachycardia through its anticholinergic effect, which may preclude its use in certain clinical situations or eliminate the need for atropine in children. Vecuronium or rocuronium may be the preferred drug for those patients in whom tachycardia may worsen their underlying clinical condition, but both drugs are much more expensive than pancuronium and require reconstitution at the time of use.

III. Tips and pearls

Pretreatment drugs are used to attenuate the adverse physiologic responses to laryngoscopy and intubation.

LOAD is the mnemonic used to stimulate recall of lidocaine, opioids, atropine, and defasciculating agents.

Ideally, any pretreatment drug should be administered 3 minutes before induction to match peak drug effect with airway manipulation. It is recommended that pretreatment drugs be given even if the time to airway manipulation is compressed or prolonged.

The following drugs should be considered as pretreatment for the specific clinical situations listed.

- Lidocaine (Xylocaine) 1.5 mg/kg IV 3 minutes before airway manipulation for patients at risk for increased ICP—medical or trauma or those with bronchospastic disease (i.e., asthma, chronic obstructive pulmonary disease, cardiac asthma)
- Fentanyl (Sublimaze) 3 mg/kg IV 3 minutes before induction for patients at risk for increased ICP—medical or trauma (tight brain), ischemic heart disease (tight heart), aneurysm or dissection, or those at risk for recurrent hemorrhage in penetrating vascular trauma but who are hemodynamically stable
- Atropine 0.02 mg/kg IV 3 minutes before induction for any child less than 10 years of age undergoing RSI with SCh, or 2 mg IV for any adult receiving a repeat dose of SCh who develops bradycardia
- Vecuronium (Norcuron), pancuronium (Pavulon), or rocuronium (Zemuron) at 10% of the normal paralyzing dose 3 minutes before induction for patients at risk for increased ICP—medical or trauma

Patients at risk for increased ICP are candidates to receive three of the four pretreatment drugs (lidocaine, fentanyl, defasciculation) and often are the most pharmacologically sophisticated intubations in the ED.

Beta-blockers (e.g., esmolol [Brevibloc]) have been shown to be beneficial in attenuating the sympathetic response to laryngoscopy. They are not effective in attenuating any rise in ICP. They may increase airway resistance, especially in patients with reactive airway disease. The main concern with beta-blockers is that they are negative inotropes; in clinical situations in which maximum cardiac output is mandatory, these agents are contraindicated. With the availability of other, more appropriate drugs (especially fentanyl), the beta-blockers have little utility in RSI in the ED.

ADDITIONAL READING

Benumof JL. Physiologic and pathophysiologic responses to intubation. In: Benumof JL, ed. *Airway management: principles and practice.* St Louis: Mosby, 1996:102–117.
Lev R, Rosen P. Prophylactic lidocaine use preintubation. *J Emerg Med* 1994;12:499–506.

Special Clinical Circumstances

17

The Pediatric Patient

Robert C. Luten

Professor of Emergency Medicine and Pediatrics,
University of Florida, Jacksonville, Florida

I. The clinical challenge

The clinical challenge is to master age-related and fundamental differences between adults and children so that the clinician can feel equally comfortable with both groups when faced with an airway emergency.

The principles of airway management in children and adults are the same. Medications used to facilitate intubation and the need for alternative airway management techniques, as well as many other aspects of the approach to airway management, are generally the same in the child and adult. There are, however, a few minor differences that must be taken into consideration in emergent airway management situations. These differences are most exaggerated in the first two years of life, after which there is a transition phase during which the pediatric airway gradually evolves into the adult airway.

This discussion will focus on the main differences between adults and children and their significance in airway management.

II. Anatomic differences

Apart from differences related to size, there are certain anatomic peculiarities of the pediatric airway. The glottic opening of the trachea is at the level of C1 in infancy. This transitions to the level of C3–4 by age 7 and to the level of C4–5 in the adult. These anatomic differences translate into a high anterior position of the glottic opening in children compared with adults. In addition, children, especially infants, possess a large tongue that occupies a relatively large portion of the oral cavity. During intubation, because of this high anterior position and the large tongue, a straight blade that elevates this distensible anatomy out of the way is preferred in children below age 3, instead of a curved blade that accomplishes this less effectively (Box 17.1).

Furthermore, children have large tonsils and adenoids that cause significant bleeding when traumatized. The angle between the epiglottis and the laryngeal opening is also more acute than that in the adult. Because of these considerations, blind nasotracheal intubation is difficult and relatively contraindicated in children under 10 years of age. Children also possess a small cricothyroid membrane. Below 3 to 4 years of age it is virtually nonexistent. For this reason needle cricothyroidotomy may be difficult, and surgical cricothyroidotomy is virtually impossible and contraindicated in infants and small children up to the age of 10 years (Chapter 11).

Although children possess a relatively anterior and high airway with the attendant difficulties in visualization of the entrance to the trachea, this phenomenon is fortunately

---

Box 17.1.   Anatomic differences between adults and children

Anatomy	Clinical significance
Large intraoral tongue occupying relatively large portion of the oral cavity	1. High anterior airway position of the glottic opening compared with that in adults
High tracheal opening: C1 in infancy versus C3–4 at age 7, C4–5 in the adult	2. Straight blade preferred over curved to push distensible anatomy out of the way to visualize the larynx
Large occiput that may cause flexion of the airway, large tongue that easily collapses against the posterior pharynx	Sniffing position is preferred. The larger occiput actually elevates the head into the sniffing position in most infants and children. A towel may be required under shoulders to elevate torso relative to head in small infants.
Cricoid ring narrowest portion of the trachea as compared with the vocal cords in the adult	1. Uncuffed tubes provide adequate seal as they fit snugly at the level of the cricoid ring.
	2. Correct tube size essential since variable expansion cuffed tubes not used
Consistent anatomic variations with age with fewer abnormal variations related to body habitus, arthritis, chronic disease	<2 years, high anterior 2 to 8, transition >8, small adult
Large tonsils and adenoids may bleed. More acute angle between epiglottis and laryngeal opening results in nasotracheal intubation attempt failures.	Blind nasotracheal intubation not indicated in children Nasotracheal intubation failure
Small cricothyroid membrane	Needle cricothyroidotomy difficult, surgical cricothyroidotomy impossible in infants and small children

---

rather consistent from one child to another, so this difficulty can be anticipated. Adults may have difficult airways related to body habitus, arthritis, or chronic disease, besides individual underlying anatomy, and are less consistent from one person to another. To review, children below the age of 2 years have higher anterior airways. Above 8 years of age the airway tends to be similar to the adult; years 2 to 8 represent a transition period. Figure 17.1 demonstrates anatomic differences particular to children.

III. **Physiologic differences**

There are many physiologic differences between children and adults, but one is of particular significance in emergency airway management: Children possess a basal oxygen consumption that is about twice that of adults. The infant metabolizes at least 6 ml of oxygen per kilogram per minute. Children also possess a proportionally smaller functional residual capacity (FRC) than that of adults. The significance of this is that the period of normoxia during apnea after an equivalent time period of preoxygenation in children is less than half that of the adult. Pulmonary pathology in critically ill patients may further reduce the ability to hyperoxygenate. It is therefore critical that these factors be taken into consideration when preoxygenating and intervening in pediatric patients. Bag-valve-mask (BVM) ventilations with cricoid pressure may be required to maintain oxygen tension during the period of apnea prior to intubation (Box 17.2).

IV. **Drug dosage, metabolism, and selection**

A significant problem in the management of pediatric emergencies is the timely and accurate delivery of medications. The use of the Broselow tape for drug dosing in children precludes many of these problems, including having to estimate weight and to remember

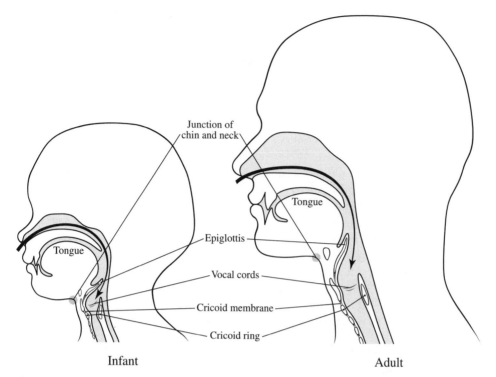

Junction of
chin and neck

Tongue

Epiglottis

Vocal cords

Cricoid membrane

Cricoid ring

Tongue

Infant

Adult

FIG. 17.1. The anatomic differences particular to children are these: 1. Higher, more anterior position for the glottic opening. (Note the relationship of the vocal cords to the chin/neck junction.) 2. Relatively larger tongue in the infant, which lies between the mouth and glottic opening. 3. Relatively larger and more floppy epiglottis in the child. 4. Cricoid ring is the narrowest portion of the pediatric airway versus the vocal cords in the adult. 5. Position and size of the cricothyroid membrane in the infant. 6. Sharper, more difficult angle for blind nasotracheal intubation. 7. Larger relative size of the occiput in the infant.

and calculate drug doses. The dose of succinylcholine in children is different from that in adults. Succinylcholine is rapidly distributed into extracellular water. Children have a larger relative volume of extracellular fluid than adults: At birth 45% of the weight is extracellular fluid water (EFW); at age 2 months, approximately 30%; at age 6 years, 20%; and at adulthood, 16% to 18%. The recommended dose of succinylcholine therefore is higher in children. In 1993 the Food and Drug Administration, in conjunction with pharmaceutical companies, revised the package labeling of succinylcholine because of reports of hyper-

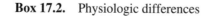

Box 17.2. Physiologic differences

Physiologic difference	Significance
Basal O_2 consumption is twice adult values (>6 ml/kg/min). Proportionally small FRC as compared with adults.	Shortened period of protection from hypoxia for equivalent preoxygenation time as compared with adults. Infants and small children often require BVM ventilation and cricoid pressure to avoid hypoxia.

kalemic cardiac arrests due to its administration to patients with previously undiagnosed neuromuscular disease. The warning went as far as saying that the drug was "contraindicated" for elective anesthesia in pediatric patients because of this concern. The wording of the warning has been softened to a more cautionary tone. However, both the initial advisory warning and the revised warning continue to recommend succinylcholine as the drug of choice for emergency or full-stomach intubation in children. Pediatric drug doses are provided in Boxes 17.3 and 17.4.

V. Equipment selection

The accompanying chart references emergency equipment needed for pediatric patients based on length (Box 17.5). Appropriate equipment can be chosen with a centimeter length measurement or with a Broselow tape. Despite best efforts (such as equipment lists or periodic checks) it is not uncommon for newborn equipment to be mixed in or placed in proximity of the smallest pediatric equipment—the pink zone. This equipment not only does not function properly, it's use may also be detrimental. Examples include the 0# Laryngoscope blade which is not long enough to allow visualization of the airway, the 250cc Newborn BVM which provides inadequate volume, and various other equipment like oral airways that can create, not alleviate obstruction, or the curved 1# Laryngoscope blade which may be difficult to use as it does not pick up the relatively large epiglottis or effectively remove the large tongue from the laryngoscopic view of the airway. A few pieces of equipment deserve mention:

A. Endotracheal tubes

The correct-sized tube for a patient can be determined by a length measurement and referring to the equipment selection chart. The formula:

$$(16 + \text{age in years}) / 4$$

Is also an accurate method of determining the correct tube size. However, it cannot be used below a year of age and is only useful if an accurate age is known, which is not always the case in an emergency. Uncuffed endotracheal tubes are recommended in the younger pediatric age groups, and cuffed tubes are used for size 5.5 mm and

---

Box 17.3.   Pediatric airway management: drug dosage, metabolism, and selection

Succinylcholine dose is higher in children: 2 mg/kg. Succinylcholine is the drug of choice for neuromuscular blockade for emergency rapid sequence intubation (RSI) in children.

A defasciculating dose of a nondepolarizer before using succinylcholine is never indicated in children < 5 years of age. Beyond 5 years of age, indications are the same as those for adults.

Always use atropine for any child under 5 years of age undergoing airway manipulation and *all* children aged ten years or less receiving succinylcholine.

Fentanyl should be used with extreme caution, as infants and small children are extremely sensitive to the respiratory depressant effect of the drug. The sympathetic blockade effect can also be detrimental if the patient is in a situation that depends on sympathetic discharge to maintain perfusion.

Lidocaine may also be effective in reactive airway disease but is not universally used in children.

The use of the Broselow tape for drug dosing children in emergencies precludes having to estimate weight or to remember and calculate drug doses.

Box 17.4.   Drugs—pediatric considerations

Drug	Dosage	Pediatric-specific comments
Premedications		
Atropine	0.02 mg/kg IV min/max dose	Prevents bradycardia 2° to airway maneuvers or succinylcholine.
Lidocaine	1.5 mg/kg IV	Head injury, asthma as for adults.
Defasciculating agent (Pan/Vecuronium)	0.01 mg/kg IV	Never <5 yr/20 kg. Above 5 yr/20 kg, use for head injury.
Fentanyl	1 to 3 µ/kg IV	In head injury. Use with extreme caution.
Induction agents		
Midazolam	0.3 mg/kg IV	Use 0.1 mg/kg if hypotensive.
Thiopental	3 to 5 mg/kg IV	Lower dose to 1 mg/kg or delete if perfusion poor.
Etomidate	0.3 mg/kg IV	
Ketamine	1 to 2 mg/kg IV 4 mg/kg IM	
Propofol	1 to 2 mg/kg IV	
Paralytics		
Succinylcholine	2 mg/kg IV	Always precede with atropine.
Pan/Vecuronium		
Defasciculation	0.01 mg/kg IV	
Paralysis	0.1 mg/kg IV	May increase to 0.3 mg/kg of vecuronium for RSI.
Rocuronium	1.0 mg/kg IV for RSI	

---

up. The rationale for this is explained earlier (Fig. 17.2). Because of the excitement of the situation, there is a tendency after intubating a patient to push the tube too far down, usually into the right mainstem bronchus. This tendency must be avoided. Insertion of the tube to an appropriate distance will avoid this. Various formulas have been proffered as aids to accomplish correct insertion length. One is the internal diameter of the tube × 3. For example, internal diameter 3.5 × 3 = 10.5 cm. To avoid recollection and calculation errors use the length-based chart, which gives tube length of insertion estimations that can be read directly from that one initial measurement.

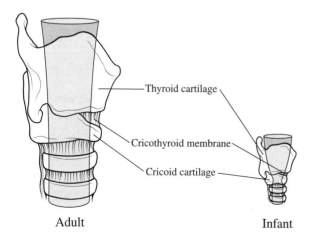

Adult   Infant

FIG. 17.2. Airway shape. Note the position of the narrowest portion of the pediatric airway, which is at the cricoid ring, creating a funnel shape, versus a straight pipe as seen in the adult, where the vocal cords form the narrowest portion. This is the rationale for using the uncuffed tube in the child; it fits snugly, unlike the cuffed tube used in the adult, which is inflated once the tube passes the cords to produce a snug fit. (Modified with permission from Cote CJ, Todres ID. The pediatric airway. In: Cote CJ, Ryan JF, Todres ID, et al, eds. *A practice of anesthesia for infants and children,* 2nd ed. Philadelphia: WB Saunders, 1993.)

Thyroid cartilage

Cricothyroid membrane

Cricoid cartilage

B. Oxygen mask

The simple rebreather mask used for most patients will only give a maximum of 35% to 60% oxygen and requires a flow of 6 to 10 L/min. A nonrebreather mask can provide approximately 75% oxygen if a flow rate of 10 to 12 L/min is used. For emergency airway management it is best to use a nonrebreather mask. A partial rebreather can give intermediate percentages of oxygen. There is no reason in an airway emergency, however, to use anything but the highest possible oxygen concentration. Some clinicians are unaware of the fact that a pediatric nonrebreather mask exists. The adult nonrebreather mask can be used for older children but is too large to be used for infants and small children.

C. Oral airways

Oral airways should only be used in patients who are unconscious. In the conscious or semiconscious patient these airways can cause vomiting. Oral airways can be selected based on the Broselow tape measurement or can be approximated by the distance from the angle of the mouth to the tragus of the ear. Insertion of oral airways will be demonstrated in the skill station.

D. Nasopharyngeal airways

Nasopharyngeal airways are ideal for use in the responsive pediatric patient. The largest nasopharyngeal airway that comfortably fits in the nasal alae should be used. However, the airway should not produce blanching of the skin at the opening nasal alae. The correct size usually goes from the tip of the nose to the tragus of the ear. Care must be taken to suction these airways regularly to avoid blockage.

E. Nasogastric tubes

Nasogastric (NG) tubes are a critical aspect of airway management in children. With BVM ventilation, the stomach often becomes distended with air, preventing effective ventilation. An NG tube should be placed soon after intubation in any patient who requires ventilation and who seems to have a tight abdomen that is preventing ventilation. Again, these may be selected using length criteria.

F. BVM equipment

For emergency airway management, the self-inflating bag-valve mask is preferred over the anesthesia ventilation bag. The BVM should have an oxygen reservoir so that when giving 10- to 15-L oxygen flow, one can obtain 90% to 95% FIO_2. The smallest bag that should be used is the 450-ml BVM. Neonatal bags that are smaller (250 ml) do not provide effective tidal volume for small infants. Many of the BVM devices have a pop-off valve. The pop-off valve is usually set around 35 to 45 cm of water and is used to prevent barotrauma by providing a release of excessive pressure generated during BVM ventilation. Because in many emergent airway situations a higher respiratory pressure is needed to ventilate a patient, the bag should either have no pop-off valve or one that is easily adjusted or occluded.

G. CO_2 detectors

Colorimetric end-tidal carbon dioxide detectors are equally useful in adults and children. A pediatric size exists for children below 15 kg. Above 15 kg the adult size should be used. Although the pediatric model will function when used with larger children, amount of resistance created when ventilating through the smaller model may preclude ability to ventilate and oxygenate the larger patient.

VI. Airway alternatives

Orotracheal intubation is the procedure of choice for emergency airway management of the pediatric patient, including those patients with potential neck injuries in whom RSI provides for rapid definitive control, to minimize the risk of aspiration and preventing movement. Nasotracheal intubation is contraindicated in children for the reasons previously discussed.

Box 17.5. Equipment selection

Length (cm) based pediatric equipment chart

	Pink	Red	Purple	Yellow	White	Blue	Orange	Green
Weight (kg)	6–7	8–9	10–11	12–14	15–18	19–23	23–31	31–41
Length (cm)	60.75–67.75	67.75–75.25	75.25–85	85–98.25	98.25–110.75	110.75–127.5	122.5–132.5	137.5–155
ET tube size (mm)	3.5	3.5	4.0	4.5	5.0	5.5	6.0 cuff	6.5 cuff
Lip-tip length (mm)	10.5	10.5	12.0	13.5	15.0	16.5	18.0	19.5
Laryngoscope	1	1	1	2	2	2	2	3
	Straight	Straight	Straight	Straight	Straight	Straight or curved	Straight or curved	Straight or curved
Suction catheter	8F	8F	8F	8–10F	10F	10F	10F	12F
Stylet	6F	6F	6F	6F	6F	14F	14F	14F
Oral airway	50 mm	50 mm	60 mm	60 mm	60 mm	70 mm	80 mm	80 mm
Nasopharyngeal Airway	14F	14F	18F	20F	22F	24F	26F	30F
Bag-valve device	Infant	Infant	Child	Child	Child	Child	Child/adult	Adult
Oxygen mask	Newborn	Newborn	Pediatric	Pediatric	Pediatric	Pediatric	Adult	Adult
Vascular access catheter/butterfly	22–24/23–25 intraosseous	22–24/23–25 intraosseous	20–22/23–25 intraosseous	18–22/21–23 intraosseous	18–22/21–23 intraosseous	18–20/21–23 intraosseous	18–20/21–22 intraosseous	16–20/18–21
Nasogastric Tube	5–8F	5–8F	8–10F	10F	10–12F	12–14F	14–18F	18F
Urinary catheter	5–8F	5–8F	8–10F	10F	10–12F	10–12F	12F	12F
Chest tube	10–12F	10–12F	16–20F	20–24F	20–24F	24–32F	24–32F	32–40F
Blood pressure cuff	Newborn/infant	Newborn/infant	Infant/child	Child	Child	Child	Child/adult	Adult
LMA†	1.5	1.5	2	2	2	2–2.5	2.5	3

Directions for use:
1. Measure patient length with centimeter tape, or with a Broselow tape.
2. Using measured length in centimeters or Broselow tape measurement, access appropriate equipment column.
3. For endotracheal tubes, oral and nasopharyngeal airways and LMAs, always select one size smaller, one size larger than the recommended size.

†Based on manufacturer's weight based guidelines

Mask Size	Patient Size
1	up to 5 kg
1.5	5–10 kg
2	10–20 kg
2.5	20–30 kg
3	Over 30 kg

Permission to reproduce with modification from Luten RC, Wears RL, Broselow J, et al. *Ann Emerg Med* 1992;21:900–904.

Box 17.6.   Alternatives for airway support

BVM Ventilation	May be the most reliable temporizing measure in children. Equipment selection, adjuncts, and good technique essential.
Orotracheal Intubation (usually with RSI)	Still the procedure of choice for emergent airway in potential cervical spine injury and most other circumstances.
Needle Cricothyroidotomy	Recommended as last resort in infants and children, but data lacking.
Laryngeal Mask	Possible alternative but requires further evaluation.
Blind Nasotracheal Intubation	Not indicated for children younger than 10 years of age.

The usual surgical alternative airway technique in adults is surgical cricothyroidotomy. Because of the minuscule size of the cricothyroid membrane in children, this procedure is at best difficult, if not contraindicated, in small children. Needle cricothyroidotomy is a recommended procedure, although there are minimal data as to its effectiveness in children. As a temporizing measure, the laryngeal mask might represent an alternative to endotracheal intubation in children. Combitubes are easy to insert, but currently there are no models for pediatric patients (Box 17.6).

VII. Initiation of Mechanical Ventilation

In pediatrics two modes of ventilation are used for emergency ventilation. For newborns and small infants, pressure-limited ventilators are traditionally used. For larger infants and older children, volume-limited ventilators are used, as in adults. One can arbitrarily set 10 kg as the upper limit for the use of pressure-limited ventilators, although volume ventilators have been used effectively in smaller children. When using pressure ventilators, the respiratory rate is initially 20 to 25 because of the small size of the infant or newborn. I/E ratios are set at 1:2. Begin with a tidal volume of 10 to 15 ml/kg. Adjust according to subsequent clinical evaluation and chest rise. PEEP should also be set at 3 to 5 cm of water and FIO_2 at 1.0. Once initial settings have been employed, it is critical that the patient be quickly reevaluated and adjustments made, because compliance and leaks can preclude adequate ventilation with initial settings. Only *clinical* determinations of adequacy should be relied on. Once the adjustments are made and the patient appears clinically to be ventilated and oxygenating, blood gas determinations or continuous pulse oximetry and ET CO_2 monitoring should be used for confirmation and further adjustments (Boxes 17.7 and 17.8).

VIII. Recommended RSI techniques for children

    1. Preparation

    2. Preoxygenation

       • Be meticulous. Children desaturate more rapidly than adults.

    3. Pretreatment

       • Atropine 0.02 mg/kg IV

       • Other pre-Rx as for condition

    4. Paralysis with induction

       • Induction agent selection as for adult: dose by length or weight.

       • Succinylcholine 2 mg/kg or by length.

Box 17.7.   Initiation of mechanical ventilation

I. Initial settings

	Pressure-limited	Volume-limited
Ventilator type	Pressure-limited	Volume-limited
Respiratory rate	20-25/minute	12–20, by age
PEEP	3–5 cm H_2O	3–5 cm H_2O
F_iO_2	1.0 (100%)	1.0 (100%)
Inspiratory time	≥0.6 sec.	≥0.6 sec.
I/E ratio	1:2	1:2

Pressure/volume settings   For pressure ventilation start with PIP of 15–20 cm H_2O. Assess chest rise and adjust to higher pressures as needed. For volume ventilation start with tidal volumes of 10–15 ml/kg. Start at lower volumes and increase to a PIP of 20–30 cm H_2O. **These are initial setting guidelines only. Assess chest rise and adjust accordingly.**

II. Evaluate clinically and make adjustments   Most patients will be ventilated with volume-cycled ventilators. Poor chest rise, poor color, decreased breath sounds require *higher* tidal volume. Check for pneumo, blocked tube. Assure tube size and position are optimal and leaks are not present. For patients ventilated with pressure-cycled ventilators, these findings may indicate the need to increase the peak inspiratory pressure.

III. Laboratory information   ABG should be performed approximately 10–15 minutes after settings are stabilized. Additional samples may be necessary after each ventilator adjustment, unless ventilatory status monitored by end-tidal CO_2 and S_{PO_2}.

Box 17.8.   Emergency pediatric airway management—practical considerations

ANATOMIC
- Anticipate high anterior glottic opening.
- Do not hyperextend the neck
- Uncuffed tubes are used in children less than 8 years old.
- Use straight blades in young children.

PHYSIOLOGIC
- Anticipate possible desaturation.

DRUGS DOSAGE AND EQUIPMENT SELECTION
- **Always** use atropine (under 10 years of age).
- Use length-based system. Do *not* use memory or do calculations.
- NG tube is an important airway adjunct in infants.
- Stock pediatric nonrebreather masks.

AIRWAY ALTERNATIVES FOR FAILED OR DIFFICULT AIRWAY
- Surgical cricothyroidotomy—contraindicated until age 10 years
- Blind NT intubation—contraindicated until age 10 years
- Combitube—only if >4 feet tall
- Needle cricothyrotomy—acceptable

5. Protection and positioning
  - Apply Sellick's maneuver
6. Placement with proof
  - Anticipate desaturation, bag-ventilate if $S_{PO_2} < 90$
  - Confirm as for adult
7. Postintubation management

ADDITIONAL READING

Berry FA, Yemen TA. Pediatric airway in health and disease. *Pediatr Anesth* 1994;41:153–180.
Cote CJ, Eavey RD, Todres ID, et al. Cricothyroid membrane puncture: oxygenation and ventilation in a dog model using an intravenous catheter. *Crit Care Med* 1988;16:615–619.
Kanter RK, Blatt S, Zimmerman J, et al. Initial mechanical ventilator settings for pediatric patients: clinical judgment in selection of tidal volume. *Am J Emerg Med* 1987;5:113.
Luten RC, Wears RL, Broselow J, et al. Length-based endotracheal tube sizing for pediatric resuscitation. *Ann Emerg Med* 1990;19:476.
Yamamoto LG, Yim GK, Britten AG. Rapid sequence anesthesia induction for emergency intubation. *Pediatr Emerg Care* 1990;6:200–213.

18

The Trauma Patient

Michael A. Gibbs

*Department of Emergency Medicine, Carolinas Medical Center,
Charlotte, North Carolina*

I. The clinical challenge

In most busy emergency departments a sizable number of intubations are performed on patients suffering major trauma. For example, 33% of patients entered in the National Emergency Airway Registry (NEAR), a multicenter airway management database that analyzed over 4,000 intubations, were victims of trauma. Timely intubation in the severely injured trauma patient improves outcome. Conversely, inadequate airway management in this patient population is the primary cause of preventable mortality.

Airway management in the trauma patient poses several unique challenges. Success requires excellent assessment skills, an understanding of the physiology of injury, a thorough knowledge of airway pharmacology, and strong leadership.

II. Rapid patient assessment

By definition, the trauma patient should be considered to have at least a potentially difficult airway. During the primary survey, one should immediately assess for

1. Injury to the face, mouth, or neck that may make the process of intubation difficult or impossible.
2. The potential for cervical spine injury and the need for in-line cervical stabilization.
3. Chest injury that may limit the patient's respiratory reserve.
4. Signs of obvious or occult hemodynamic instability that can be worsened or unmasked by some of the pharmacologic agents used for rapid sequence intubation (RSI).
5. The presence of traumatic brain injury, which may alter airway management decision making and drug selection.

This information will be forthcoming during the primary and secondary survey. Some of the essentials can be rapidly determined at the bedside in 10 to 20 seconds. As soon as the patient is moved to the stretcher in the trauma room, asking the following four questions will provide rapid assessment:

"What is your name?"

"Are you having trouble breathing?"

"Can you move your toes?"

"Where do you hurt?"

Answers to these questions will immediately help establish the patient's level of consciousness and Glasgow Coma Score (GCS), elicit signs of upper-airway obstruction or labored breathing, assess the integrity of the spinal cord, and focus on the predominant anatomic sites of injury.

Next, examine the airway carefully for edema, intraoral bleeding, or a foreign body. Although it is important to determine the patient's ability to handle secretions, "testing the gag reflex" is not recommended, as this maneuver may precipitate vomiting and worsen intracranial hypertension. An assessment of the patient's hemodynamic status and physical examination of the torso will give additional information crucial to the airway management plan. Remember to document a brief neurologic examination (GCS, pupillary response and symmetry, and level of motor activity in each of the four limbs) before giving neuromuscular blocking agents. This information will assist the neurosurgeon with subsequent management of the patient with traumatic brain injury.

In tandem with the primary and secondary survey, preparation for airway management should be ongoing:

1. Be sure the patient is adequately monitored (HR, BP, S_pO_2).
2. Secure at least two large-bore intravenous catheters.
3. Assemble all airway equipment and drugs.
4. Specifically assess the patient for a difficult airway and formulate a backup airway plan, should RSI not succeed or not be felt desirable.
5. Assign specific tasks to all team members (i.e., designate members to give drugs, stabilize the spine, hold cricoid pressure, assist with intubation). This will help organize the trauma resuscitation and maintain control of the room.

III. Issues in trauma airway management

A. Cervical spine injury

All severely injured blunt-trauma patients have cervical injury until proven otherwise. In the vast majority of cases the patient will be immobilized by prehospital providers in the field. Although this is essential to prevent further spinal injury, it can create several problems as well. Intoxicated or head-injured patients typically become agitated and difficult to control when strapped down on a back board. Physical and chemical restraint may be required. Aspiration is a significant risk in the supine patient with traumatic brain injury or intraoral bleeding. In this position ventilation may be impaired, especially in the presence of pulmonary injury. High-flow oxygen should be provided to all patients, and suction must be immediately available.

If urgent airway management is needed, *do not* waste time getting a cross-table lateral cervical spine x-ray prior to intubation. This single view is inadequate to exclude injury, with a sensitivity of 85% at best. Waiting for the x-ray will waste precious time and give the operator a false sense of security when the film is interpreted as "normal." Instead, assume all patients have cervical injury and maintain in-line stabilization at all times. This should also be documented in the medical record (e.g., "in-line stabilization maintained during RSI . . .").

Much debate has centered around the safety of oral intubation in the presence of cervical spine injury. Practitioners and scholars alike were deeply divided on this issue. One theory argued that blunt injury could create an instability in the cervical spine and that manipulation of the airway during direct laryngoscopy might cause movement of the unstable elements, thus resulting in spinal cord injury. This argument, although largely theoretical, was widely accepted and was one of the principal factors in the adoption of blind nasotracheal intubation as the airway maneuver of choice in the multiply injured blunt-trauma patient. If nasotracheal intubation was impossible, surgical cricothyroidotomy was recommended. The countervailing position was that oral endotracheal intubation could be safely performed even in the presence of cervical spine injury, provided that proper technique was used and strict attention was paid to meticulous immobilization of the cervical spine throughout the process of intubation. Although no definitive study has demonstrated the safety of oral intubation in the presence of cervical spine injury, an increasing body of literature argues in favor of the safety of this maneuver. Several large series and one cineflouroscopic study show no evidence that properly performed RSI with in-line cervical immobilization presents any hazard to the patient, even in the presence of proven cervical spine injury. Oral endotracheal intubation of the blunt-trauma patient with suspected or proven cervical spine injury is safe and is the airway maneuver of choice, provided:

1. Laryngoscopy and intubation are performed in a gentle, atraumatic manner. RSI is the preferred technique, as it allows for immediate airway control and eliminates the risk of patient movement during laryngoscopy.
2. Precise cervical immobilization is maintained throughout the intubation sequence. This requires the presence of a second individual, whose sole responsibility is manual immobilization of the spine. Ideally, this person should stand at the side of the bed rather than at the head of the bed to give the intubator unimpeded access to the airway.

When the assessment indicates that intubation will be difficult or impossible, an alternative technique should be considered. The technique employed in this situation (e.g., "awake" laryngoscopy with sedation, fiberoptic intubation, lighted-stylet intubation, blind nasotracheal intubation, cricothyroidotomy) will depend on the clinical scenario and the experience of the operator (see chapters 3 and 5).

B. Shock

Patients suffering significant injury may have obvious or occult hypotension from many different sources. Victims of blunt multisystem trauma are especially vulnerable. Shock in this patient population can be broadly classified as hemorrhagic (e.g., external, intrathoracic, intraabdominal, retroperitoneal, long-bone) or nonhemorrhagic (e.g., tension pneumothorax, pericardial tamponade, myocardial contusion, spinal shock). A diligent search for the primary source (s) of hypotension must begin at once. Remember that patients on the verge of cardiovascular collapse often maintain a "normal" blood pressure, especially if they are young.

Several of the agents used for RSI may cause significant myocardial depression and vasodilatation that will worsen shock in the hypovolemic patient. This is especially true for the barbiturates (e.g., thiopental) and the benzodiazepines (e.g., midazolam). Both drugs are contraindicated in the hemodynamically unstable patient and should be used with caution even in "normotensive" patients at risk. Although fentanyl has an excellent hemodynamic profile, it can significantly worsen shock in patients who are dependent on sympathetic drive (as are all shock patients) because of its sympathetic blocking activity. If RSI is planned, etomidate, which possesses a favorable hemodynamic profile, is the preferred induction agent. Ketamine is also an excellent choice, provided there is no evidence of intracranial hypertension (see chapter 15).

C. Traumatic brain injury

Maintenance of cerebral oxygenation and perfusion are fundamental goals during the initial resuscitation of the patient with severe head injury. Hypoxemia and hypotension should be avoided at all costs, as either will worsen outcome. It has been demonstrated that a single episode of hypoxia (PO_2 < 60 mmHg), or hypotension (blood pressure [BP] < 90 mmHg) increases mortality in the brain-injured patient by 150%. Provision of a stable airway and aggressive hemodynamic resuscitation should be the priorities of initial care. The American Association of Neurologic Surgery recommends intubation for all patients with a GCS of 8 or less . In head-injured patients with higher GCS scores, the threshold should be lowered if other severe injuries exist, if the patient must leave the safety of the ED (e.g., for computed tomography [CT] scan, angiogram, or transfer), or if the patient is clearly deteriorating.

In the patient with traumatic brain injury and impaired cerebral autoregulation, stimulation of the airway during laryngoscopy may worsen intracranial hypertension. This is believed to be mediated by a direct response to laryngoscopy as well as an indirect sympathetically mediated response. RSI is the procedure of choice for airway control in the brain-injured patient. The technique should be focused on methods to attenuate the potential rise in ICP that accompanies laryngoscopic examination. Several drugs may be used to attenuate this physiologic response. Pretreatment with lidocaine will block the direct response and should be employed in all patients with brain injury. Pretreatment with fentanyl attenuates the indirect response and should also be considered, provided the patient is hemodynamically stable. Etomidate, a drug that protects the brain while maintaining stable hemodynamics, is the preferred induction agent. Although thiopental provides excellent cerebroprotection, it is also a potent myocardial depressant and vasodilator, and must be used with caution. Although this is controversial, ketamine should probably not be used in patients with brain injury, because it may increase ICP. Head injury management is discussed in detail in Chapter 19.

D. Disrupted airway anatomy

The patient who presents with distorted airway anatomy secondary to maxillofacial trauma presents a significant challenge. The very condition that may mandate intubation will also render it much more difficult and prone to failure. Direct airway injury may be the result of the following:

1. Maxillofacial trauma
2. Blunt or penetrating anterior neck trauma
3. Smoke inhalation
4. Caustic ingestion

In cases of distorted anatomy, the approach must be one that minimizes the potential for catastrophic deterioration. Although some argue in favor of a period of expectant observation, waiting for the nearly obstructed airway to become completely obstructed can be disastrous. In many cases expansion of a deep hematoma may not be clinically obvious.

A careful approach must be planned, taking into account the expertise of the physician(s) in the department and in the hospital, the equipment at hand, the need for transfer, the urgency of the need for surgery, the need for diagnostic studies, and many other factors. If there is a theme that unifies the approach to this type of airway problem, it is "plan ahead." The optimal approach for airway management will vary, depending on the clinical scenario. In patients with signs of significant airway compromise (e.g., stridor, drooling, respiratory distress, expanding neck hematoma), the risk of using neuromuscular blockade is high, and it may be most appropriate to attempt awake intubation with sedation or proceed directly to a surgical airway. When symptoms are modest but elective intubation is still indicated (e.g., before interfacility transport), a combined approach may be used, in which an awake technique is used to ensure adequacy of laryngoscopy; then RSI is used for the actual intubation. This can be accomplished by gentle laryngoscopy or nasopharyngoscopy.

E. Chest trauma

Chest injury results from a variety of conditions and impairs ventilation and oxygenation. These conditions include pneumothorax, hemothorax, flail chest, pulmonary contusion, and open chest wounds. Preoxygenation may be impossible in these patients, and rapid desaturation may occur following paralysis. In addition, the positive pressure delivered via the endotracheal tube may convert a simple pneumothorax to a tension pneumothorax. Patients with a known or suspected pneumothorax should have tube thoracostomy performed before RSI if their clinical status permits. Insertion of the chest tube may restore hemodynamic stability and oxygenation, thus making the intubation safer. If the patient requires immediate intubation, the chest may be vented with a catheter, and a chest tube should be inserted immediately after intubation.

IV. **Paralysis versus rapid tranquilization of the combative trauma patient**
The combative trauma patient presents a series of conflicting problems. The causes of combative behavior in the trauma patient are numerous and include head injury, drug or ethanol intoxication, preexisting medical conditions (diabetes in particular), hypoxemia, shock, anxiety, personality disorder, and others. The priority is to control the patient rapidly so that potentially life-threatening injuries can be identified and corrected. Controversy exists as to whether such patients ought to undergo rapid tranquilization with a neuroleptic agent or sedative or whether immediate intubation with neuromuscular blockade is appropriate. Rapid tranquilization using haloperidol or droperidol is well established as a safe and effective means for gaining control of the combative trauma patient. Haloperidol can be used intravenously in 5- to 10-mg increments every 3 to 5 minutes until a clinical response is achieved. Extensive literature supports the safety of this approach. Alternatively, droperidol, a similar neuroleptic agent, can be used in doses of 2.5 to 10 mg intravenously or intramuscularly. Opioids, such as morphine or fentanyl, should not be used because of their profound respiratory-depressant effects.

The decision to employ rapid tranquilization rather than RSI with neuromuscular blockade should rest on the nature of the patient's presentation and injuries. If intubation is indicated on the basis of injuries identified and if the patient is in need of control, then immediate intubation is indicated. If the patient is presenting primarily with control problems and does not appear to be seriously injured, rapid tranquilization is appropriate. In many situations the decision will not be clear-cut. When a diagnostic dilemma exists, it is most prudent to assume the worst and not dismiss profoundly altered mentation as merely the consequence of inebriation. Always protect the patient.

V. **Use of neuromuscular blocking agents in trauma patients**
Advantages of RSI in the trauma patient include the following:
   1. The most rapid attainment of a definitive airway
   2. Ability to perform gentle controlled laryngoscopy in cases of head injury or suspected cervical spine injury
   3. Control of the combative, severely injured patient
   4. Facilitation of specific diagnostic and therapeutic procedures
   5. A higher success rate and lower complication rate than other available methods

Succinylcholine has been the mainstay of RSI in the ED. The advantages of succinylcholine include its rapid onset and brief duration of action. Concerns about causing hyperkalemia in patients with burns or crush injury are not relevant in the acute setting, as this does not occur for at least 48 hours. Succinylcholine has also been implicated in the elevation of intracranial pressure in the patient with traumatic brain injury. This can be mitigated by appropriate use of a competitive neuromuscular blocking agent in a "defasciculating" dose before administration of succinylcholine. Recently, rapacuronium, an ultra short-acting competitive neuromuscular blocking agent, has been approved. Competitive blockade has been advocated for use in RSI, however, although the onset of rocuronium is as rapid as that of succinylcholine, its duration of action is significantly longer. Rocuronium should be used in those circumstances in which succinylcholine is contraindicated.

VI. **The difficult trauma airway**
An essential part of the "preparation" phase of RSI is the formulation of a rescue plan if RSI fails. This is especially important in the trauma setting, when facial or upper-airway

trauma may make intubation difficult or impossible. All clinicians using neuromuscular blocking agents should be proficient with surgical airway management. Because the technique is invasive and used infrequently, even seasoned emergency physicians may have limited or no experience with surgical cricothyroidotomy, and it is important to review the procedure often, at least mentally.

A. Tips and pearls

A rapid bedside assessment should help you anticipate the difficult airway.

Essentials of the physical examination should elicit clinical evidence of spinal injury, traumatic brain injury, occult hypovolemia, direct airway trauma, and pulmonary dysfunction.

All blunt-trauma patients have injury to the cervical spine until proven otherwise. In-line stabilization should be performed and documented.

The priority in the initial management of the patient with traumatic brain injury is to maintain adequate central nervous system perfusion and oxygenation at all costs.

In the patient with direct injury to the airway, the clinician must always have an immediate plan (and the equipment) for airway rescue should RSI fail.

Many of the drugs used for RSI (the benzodiazepines and barbiturates in particular) may precipitate hypotension in the hypovolemic patient.

Oral endotracheal intubation using RSI is the airway maneuver of choice in most trauma patients. A well-thought-out management plan that takes into account the patient's known or suspected injuries and hemodynamic status will help the clinician rapidly develop and orchestrate an individualized airway management plan. During the often chaotic environment of a trauma resuscitation, consistency, calmness, effective reasoning, communication, and leadership are the ingredients for success.

ADDITIONAL READING

American Association of Neurologic Surgeons Guidelines for the management of severe head injury: The integration of brain-specific treatments into the initial resuscitation of the severe head trauma patient. *J Neurosurg* 1996;15:653.

Blahd WH, Iserson KV, Bjelland JC. Efficacy of the posttraumatic cross table lateral view of the cervical spine. *J Emerg Med* 1985;2:243.

Ebert JP, Pearson JD, Gelman S, et al. Circulatory response to laryngoscopy: the comparative response of placebo, fentanyl and esmolol. *Can J Anaesth* 1989;36:301.

Esposito TJ, Sanddal ND, Hansen JD, et al. Analysis of preventable trauma deaths and inappropriate trauma care in a rural state. *J Trauma* 1995;39:955.

MacGillivray RG, Rocke DA, Mahomedy AE, et al. Midazolam for induction of anaesthesia in patients with limited cardiac reserves: a comparison with etomidate. *S Afr Med J* 1988;73:101.

Shaffer MA, Doris PE. Limitation of the cross table lateral view in detecting cervical spine injuries: A retrospective analysis. *Ann Emerg Med* 1981;10:508–513.

Shatney CH, Brunner RD, Nguyen TQ. The safety of orotracheal intubation in patients with unstable cervical spine fracture or high spinal cord injury. *Am J Surg* 1995;170:676.

Stocchetti N, Furlan A, Volta F. Hypoxemia and arterial hypotension at the accident scene in head injury. *J Trauma* 1996;40:764.

Streitwieser DR, Knopp R, Wales LR, et al. Accuracy of standard radiographic views in detecting cervical spine fractures. *Ann Emerg Med* 1983;12:538.

Trupka A, Waydhas C, NastKolb D, et al. Early intubation in severely injured patients. *Eur J Emerg Med* 1995;1:1.

Walls RM. Airway management in the blunt trauma patient: how important is the cervical spine. *Can J Surg* 1992;35:27.

Walls RM. Cricothyroidotomy. *Emerg Med Clin North Am* 1993;11:53.

Walls RM, Wolfe R, Rosen R. Fools rush in? Airway management in penetrating neck trauma [editorial]. *J Emerg Med* 1993;11:479–482.

19

Increased Intracranial Pressure

Ron M. Walls* and Michael F. Murphy†

*Chairman, Department of Emergency Medicine, Brigham and Women's Hospital,
Associate Professor of Medicine, Division of Emergency Medicine, Harvard Medical School,
Boston, Massachusetts; †Departments of Emergency Medicine and Anaesthesiology,
Queen Elizabeth II Health Sciences Centre, Dalhousie University, Halifax, Nova Scotia

I. The clinical challenge

Patients with increased intracranial pressure (ICP) present a particular clinical challenge. The ICP increase is a direct threat to the viability and function of the brain. Many of the techniques used for airway management have the potential to further increase ICP, thus compounding the problem. Many of these patients are the victims of multiple trauma and present with hypotension, thus limiting the choice of agents and techniques available. This chapter will provide the basis for an understanding of the problems of increased ICP and the optimal methods of airway management in this patient group.

When increased ICP occurs as a result of injury or medical catastrophe, it must be presumed that autoregulation is lost. Autoregulation is the ability to regulate blood flow to the brain over a wide range of mean arterial blood pressures. In general, ICP is maintained through a mean arterial blood pressure range of 80–180 mm/hg. When increased ICP has developed, autoregulation often, but not always, has been lost. In this setting, excessively high or excessively low blood pressure could aggravate brain injury. Hypotension is especially harmful, and must be avoided, if possible.

Cerebral perfusion pressure (CPP) is the driving force for blood flow to the brain, and is measured by the difference between the mean arterial blood pressure (MAP) and the ICP. Expressed as a formula,

$$CPP = MAP - ICP$$

It is clear from this formula that excessive decreases in MAP during intubation would be undesirable in the context of elevated ICP. It might also appear that increases in MAP, almost without bound, would be beneficial because of the increase in the driving pressure for oxygenation of brain tissue. However, because of the loss of autoregulation, increases in MAP can translate directly to increases in ICP. Thus, not only is the driving gradient for CPP increased, but the absolute ICP is increased as well. Accordingly, it is important to try to maintain mean arterial blood pressure in the range of 100–110 mmHg to optimize cerebral perfusion and to minimize absolute ICP.

There are a number of confounding elements that may increase ICP during airway management. These are:

A. Reflex sympathetic response to laryngoscopy (RSRL)

This reflex is stimulated by the rich sensory innervation of the supraglottic larynx. Use of the laryngoscope or attempted placement of an endotracheal tube results in a significant afferent discharge which causes sympathetic activity including the release of catecholamines from the adrenal glands. Longer, more aggressive attempts at laryngoscopy result in greater and more prolonged sympathetic nervous system stimulation. This catecholamine surge leads to increased heart rate and blood pressure, potentially aggravating the ICP problems as described above if autoregulation is impaired. It is desirable to mitigate this RSRL. In addition to using a gentle, controlled technique, the RSRL can be effectively blunted by administration of either a beta blocker or of one of the synthetic opioids, such as fentanyl. In general, in these emergency department patients, administration of a beta blocker is not desirable. Therefore, the recommendation is to administer fentanyl as a pretreatment drug in patients with elevated ICP. Although a full sympathetic blocking dose of fentanyl is 9 to 13 µ/kg, the recommended dose of fentanyl for this purpose in emergency department patients is 3 µ/kg. This should be administered as a single pretreatment dose over 30 to 60 seconds. This technique permits effective mitigation of the RSRL with greatly reduced chances of apnea or hypoventilation before sedation and paralysis.

B. Reflex ICP response to laryngoscopy

Laryngoscopy may also increase the ICP by a direct reflex mechanism not mediated by blood pressure or heart rate. Insertion of the laryngoscope or endotracheal tube may itself further elevate ICP, even if the RSRL is blunted. It is desirable to blunt this ICP response to laryngoscopy. It has been shown that the administration of lidocaine in a dose of 1.5 mg/kg intravenously effectively blunts the ICP response to endotracheal suctioning and laryngeal stimulation. Lidocaine may also reduce ICP absolutely. Therefore, in patients with elevated ICP, lidocaine should be administered as a pretreatment drug in the dose of 1.5 mg/kg intravenously 3 minutes before succinylcholine (SCh) to mitigate the ICP response to laryngoscopy and intubation.

C. CHOICE OF NEUROMUSCULAR BLOCKING AGENT

1. ICP response to Succinylcholine (SCh)

SCh itself appears capable of causing an increase in ICP. Studies have shown that this increase is temporally related to the presence of fasciculations in the patient, but is not the result of synchronized muscular activity leading to increased venous pressure. Rather, there appears to be a complex reflex mechanism originating in the muscle spindle and ultimately resulting in an elevation of ICP. One recent study challenged the claim that SCh causes an elevation of ICP and SCh remains the drug of choice for management of patients with elevated ICP because of its rapid onset and short duration. Studies have shown that administration of a full paralyzing dose of a competitive neuromuscular blocker before the SCh completely abolishes the ICP rise associated with SCh. It has also been shown that the administration of a small "defasciculating" dose of a competitive neuromuscular blocker, approximately one-tenth of the paralyzing dose, effectively blunts this intracranial response to SCh. Therefore, when SCh is used to intubate patients with suspected ICP increase, a defasciculating dose of a competitive neuromuscular blocker, such as 0.01 mg/kg of pancuronium or vecuronium, should be administered during the pretreatment phase of the rapid sequence intubation. Fasciculation can also be reduced by administration of a small dose of SCh (0.2mg/kg) 3 minutes before the full dose, but the effect of this on ICP, if any, is not known.

2. Alternatives to SCh

Unlike SCh, non-depolarizing (competitive) neuromuscular blocking agents do not cause elevation of ICP, although ICP increase will still be stimulated by the act of intubation. Therefore, it may be preferable to use these agents instead of SCh for intubation in patients with raised ICP. Rapacuronium and rocuronium are the competitive agents most suited to this strategy due to their rapid onset and limited duration of action. In addition, when a competitive agent is used, no "defasciculating" dose is needed, thus simplifying the intubation sequence. Both rapacuronium and rocuronium have rapid onset, but one potential drawback may be the duration of paralysis, particularly if the airway cannot be secured. With rapacuronium, however, administration of reversal agents can result in restoration of spontaneous ventilation within 10 minutes in the unlikely circumstance that the patient can be neither intubated nor successfully oxygenated with bag and mask. The competitive neuromuscular blocking agents and their reversal are discussed in Chapter 14, and use of these agents for RSI is in Chapter 7.

D. Choice of induction agent

Because of the elevated ICP, it is important to choose an induction agent that, at the least, will not make matters worse. Ideally, one would like to choose an induction agent that is capable of reducing ICP, improving or maintaining CPP and providing some cerebral protective effect. Sodium thiopental is an ultra short-acting barbiturate induction agent. Thiopental confers some cerebroprotective effect because it decreases the basal metabolic rate of oxygen utilization of the brain ($CMRO_2$). This can be likened to decreasing myocardial oxygen demand in the ischemic heart. In addition, sodium thiopental decreases cerebral blood flow, thus decreasing ICP. This combination of characteristics, the decrease in ICP and the decrease in $CMRO_2$ make thiopental a desirable agent for use in patients with elevated ICP. However, thiopental is a potent venodilator and negative inotrope. Therefore, it has a tendency to cause significant hypotension, even in relatively hemodynamically stable patients. In the hemodynamically unstable patient, this hypotensive effect can be profound. Hypotension significantly increases mortality in acute, severe head injury. Therefore, although thiopental is a desirable agent for management of patients with elevated ICP, its hemodynamic instability relegates it to an alternative role, with etomidate being the agent of choice.

Etomidate is a short-acting imidazole derivative that has a similar profile of activity to thiopental, but without the tendency to cause hemodynamic compromise. In fact, etomidate is the most hemodynamically stable of all commonly used induction agents. Its ability to decrease $CMRO_2$ and ICP in a manner analogous to that of sodium thiopental and its remarkable hemodynamic stability make it the drug of choice for patients with elevated ICP. (See Chapter 15.)

II. Approach to airway management

Rapid sequence intubation is the preferred method for patients with suspected elevated ICP because its high success rate and low complication rate, and because of the need to control adverse reflexes, hemodynamics, and ventilation. Following appropriate assessment and preparation as described in Chapter 2, the sequence in box 19-1 is recommended for patients with elevated ICP.

III. Initiating mechanical ventilation

Mechanical ventilation in the patient with elevated ICP should be predicated upon two principles: 1) optimal oxygenation, and 2) avoidance of ventilation mechanics (e.g., positive end-expiratory pressure [PEEP], high peak inspiratory pressure [PIP]) that would increase venous congestion in the brain.

Controlled hyperventilation to a $Paco_2$ of approximately 30 mmHg was formerly recommended for the early management of elevated ICP. It was believed that reduction in $Paco_2$ tensions in the brain leads to vasoconstriction, decreased cerebral blood flow, and

---

Box 19.1.   RSI sequence for patients with elevated ICP

Time	**Action** (seven Ps)
Zero minus 10 minutes	**P**reparation
Zero minus 5 minutes	**P**reoxygenation
Zero minus 3 minutes	**P**retreatment:
	Lidocaine 1.5 mg/kg IV
	Vecuronium 0.01 mg/kg IV
	Fentanyl 3 µ/kg (over one minute)
Zero	**P**aralysis with Induction:
	Etomidate 0.3 µg/kg IV
	SCh 1.5 mg/kg IV
Zero plus 20 to 30 seconds	**P**rotection and positioning
Zero plus 45 seconds	**P**lacement with proof: intubate, confirm placement
Zero plus 60 seconds	**P**ostintubation management

---

therefore decreased ICP. Further declines in $Paco_2$ below 30 mmHg were not recommended because it was felt the vasoconstriction may become so severe as to compromise cerebral circulation. The scientific basis for controlled hyperventilation has not been clearly established with outcome studies, and the balance of data would appear to argue against it. The 1995 report of the Brain Trauma Foundation challenges the use of hyperventilation as a therapy for increased ICP, and recommends that patients be ventilated in such a way as to promote normocapnia. Hyperventilation to a $Paco_2$ of 30 mmHg should only be used when osmotic agents and CSF drainage are not effective in managing an acute rise in ICP accompanied by patient deterioration. Normal initial ventilation parameters include a ventilatory rate of approximately 10 to 12 breaths per minute with a tidal volume of approximately 10 cc/kg. This would result in an approximately physiologic $Paco_2$ level in the normal patient. Therefore, the initial ventilator settings should maintain tidal volume at 10 to 12 cc/kg and the ventilatory rate at 10 breaths per minute. Initial inspired fraction of oxygen (F_iO_2) should be 1.0 (100%). F_iO_2 can later be decreased according to pulse oximetry, as long as 100% oxygen saturation is maintained. Carbon dioxide tension can be followed with arterial blood gases or capnography, the first assessment of which should occur approximately 10 minutes after initiation of steady state mechanical ventilation. In addition, long-term sedation and paralysis should be undertaken to permit effective controlled mechanical ventilation and other necessary interventions. A full paralyzing dose of a competitive neuromuscular blocking agent, such as pancuronium 0.1 mg/kg or vecuronium 0.1 mg/kg should be given, along with an initial dose of 0.2 mg/kg of diazepam. Subsequently, doses of approximately ⅓ of the initial dose of both agents should be given if the patient shows evidence of regaining consciousness, increased sympathetic activity, or initiating motor movement.

IV. Tips and pearls

Rapid sequence intubation is clearly the desired method for tracheal intubation in patients with suspected elevation of ICP. The technique allows control of various adverse effects and optimal control of ventilation after intubation. However, the use of neuromuscular blockade in patients with potential neurologic deficit carries the responsibility of performing a detailed neurologic evaluation on the patient prior to initiation of neuromuscular blockade. The patient's ability to interact with the surroundings, spontaneous motor movement, response to deep pain, response to voice, localization, pupillary reflexes, and other pertinent neurological details must be assessed carefully prior to administration of neuro-muscular blockade. The careful recording of these findings will be invaluable for the on-going evaluation of the patient.

If the patient's ventilatory status is severely compromised by the head injury, positive pressure ventilation with bag and mask may be required throughout the intubation sequence. In such circumstances, one is trading off the increased risk of aspiration against the hazard of inadequate oxygenation and rising $Paco_2$ during the intubation sequence. When such a tradeoff arises, it should be resolved in favor of oxygenation over the risk of aspiration.

ADDITIONAL READING

Brain Trauma Foundation. *Guidelines for the management of severe head injury*. New York: The Brain Trauma Foundation, 1995.

Hoff JT. Special Book review and synopsis: guidelines for the management of severe head injury. *J Trauma Injury Infection and Critical Care* 1996;40:1048–1050. (An excellent summary of the Brain Trauma Foundation guidelines)

Murphy MF. Elevated intracranial pressure. In: Dailey R, ed. *The airway: emergency management*. St Louis: Mosby, 1992.

Walls RM. Airway management. *Emerg Med Clin North Am* 1993;11:53–60.

Walls RM. Airway management. In: Rosen P, ed. *Emergency medicine: concepts and clinical practice*. St Louis: Mosby, 1998.

Walls RM. Rapid sequence intubation in head trauma. *Ann Emerg Med* 1993;22:1008–1013.

20

Asthma and COPD

Robert E. Schneider

Carolinas Medical Center, Department of Emergency Medicine,
Charlotte, North Carolina

The greatest challenge in intubating and managing the patient with asthma or chronic obstructive pulmonary disease (COPD) is that the patient's clinical condition may worsen after intubation, when the patient may prove extremely difficult to ventilate and may be hemodynamically unstable. Thus the decision to intubate must be made carefully and the technique must be chosen to facilitate the best possible outcome.

I. Asthma

The asthma patient often presents one of the most difficult airway cases encountered in the emergency department. A succinct, well-focused, timely history and physical examination, together with clinical judgment, are essential in appropriate decision making. An altered level of consciousness signifies progressive hypoxia or hypercarbia that dictates immediate intervention with high-flow oxygen and rapid sequence intubation (RSI). If the patient can speak, it is imperative to ask about significant comorbid illness, especially cardiac disease, pulmonary infections, duration of symptoms, and whether the patient has ever required intubation. If intubation has been required in the past, when was the last time and, most important, how did that episode compare with the current exacerbation? If the patient states that this current event is comparable to the intubation event, one must be prepared to move quickly and secure the airway if the patient fatigues or fails to respond to initial aggressive beta$_2$-agonist and anticholinergic therapy, 100% oxygen, and steroids. The diaphoretic asthmatic patient who cannot speak full sentences, appears anxious, or is sitting upright and leaning forward to augment his or her inspiratory effort must not be left unattended until stabilized and clearly improving.

Standard initial management of acute severe asthma exacerbations includes continuous beta$_2$-agonist inhalation therapy (albuterol [Ventolin] 15 to 20 mg/h) for reversal of dynamic bronchospasm and intravenous (methylprednisolone [Solumedrol] 125 mg) for the treatment of the consistent inflammatory component. If the patient is severely bronchospastic or cannot comply with a nebulized treatment, then subcutaneous terbutaline (Brethine) 0.2 to 0.5 mg may be administered immediately. The addition of intravenous terbutaline is controversial and does not seem to augment clinical improvement but, if selected, should be initiated in the adult at 4 µg/kg over 10 minutes followed by a continuous infusion of 0.04 to 0.2 µg/kg/min; and in the child at 10 µg/kg over 30 minutes followed by a continuous infusion of 0.1 µg/kg/min. Intravenous albuterol (Salbutamol) can be administered at 3 µg/kg over 10 minutes followed by an infusion of 0.04 to 0.2 µg/kg/min in the adult. The subsequent addition of inhaled ipratropium bromide (Atrovent) or gly-copyrrolate (Robinul), intravenous anticholinergic agents (atropine or glycopyrrolate [Robinul]), intravenous magnesium sulfate, intravenous infusions of ketamine (Ketalar), or use of heliox is controversial. There is no role for intravenous aminophylline. (The reader is referred to an excellent review of this topic by Jagoda, Shepherd, Spevitz, et al.)

Despite this vast array of treatment modalities, 1% to 3% of acute severe asthma exacerbations will require intubation. These patients are usually fatigued and have reduced functional residual capacity, so it is very difficult, if not impossible, to preoxygenate them optimally. With the rapid administration of any drug, including ketamine or opioids, the patient will quickly lose respiratory drive, rapidly desaturate, and most likely become apneic, depending on individual physical reserve. Because most of these patients have been struggling for hours to promote breathing and have failed, they have little, if any, residual physical reserve and mechanical ventilation will be required. This argues against awake intubation techniques, such as nasotracheal intubation, which take longer, exacerbate hypoxemia, and are unpleasant for the patient.

Thus the single most important tenet in managing the status asthmaticus patient who requires intubation is to take total control of the airway early. This can only be accomplished through RSI that yields a totally paralyzed patient, optimum intubating conditions, and quickly and successfully passing the largest possible endotracheal tube while minimizing the possibility of epistaxis, laryngospasm, increased bronchospasm, vomiting and aspiration, and failed intubation that often occur when nasal intubation is attempted by even the most experienced intubator. The most experienced laryngoscopist present should be immediately prepared to intubate the asthmatic patient because failed laryngoscopy will result in a patient who will be very difficult, if not impossible, to oxygenate adequately by bag and mask.

If the patient appears most comfortable sitting upright, maintain the upright position. All patients with reactive airway disease or obstructive lung disease should be pretreated with 1.5 mg/kg of intravenous lidocaine (Xylocaine) 3 minutes before induction to attenuate the respiratory response to airway manipulation. Ketamine (Ketalar) is the induction agent of choice in the asthmatic patient. Ketamine stimulates the release of catecholamines and has a direct bronchial smooth muscle relaxing effect that may be important in this clinical setting. Ketamine 1.5 mg/kg is given intravenously immediately before the administration of 1.5 mg/kg of succinylcholine (Anectine). Both of these drugs should be administered to the patient in their position of comfort, often sitting upright. Once the patient loses consciousness, apply cricoid pressure, place the patient supine, and perform laryngoscopy and intubation, preferably with an 8.0- to 9.0-mm endotracheal tube. The large size of the endotracheal tube is important to decrease resistance and facilitate aggressive pulmonary toilette.

Once the patient has been successfully intubated and proper tube position has been confirmed, continuous sedation and paralysis for at least the next 4 to 6 hours with an appropriate benzodiazepine (e.g. diazepam [Valium] 15 to 20 mg IV), and a competitive muscle relaxant will prevent asynchronous respirations, promote total relaxation of fatigued respiratory muscles, decrease the production of carbon dioxide, and allow optimum ventilator settings, all of which are mandatory in the initial management of the critically ill asthmatic patient. Additional ketamine as well as continuous in-line albuterol and other pharmacologic adjuncts may also be given.

A. Mechanical ventilation

All asthmatic patients have obstructed airways and dynamic alveolar hyperinflation with varying amounts of end-expiratory residual intraalveolar gas and pressure (auto-peak end-expiratory pressure [auto-PEEP] or intrinsic PEEP). Elevations in auto-PEEP increase the risk for baro/volutrauma. Reversal of airflow obstruction and decompression of end-expiratory filled alveoli are the primary goals of early mechanical ventilation in the asthmatic. The former requires continuous in-line nebulization with increasingly higher doses of beta$_2$-agonists until reversal is objectively measured (decrease in peak and plateau airway pressures) or unacceptable side effects are produced. Safe, uncomplicated alveolar decompression requires prolonged expiratory time (I/E of 1:3 to 1:5), knowledge of basic ventilator language, and an understanding of how to set and then manipulate ventilator settings, depending on the patient's response to ongoing therapy. A detailed discussion of ventilation parameters can be found in Chapter 29. This discussion will focus on the asthmatic patient.

Initial tidal volume should be reduced to 6 to 8 ml/kg to avoid barotrauma and air trapping.

The ventilation rate should be determined in conjunction with the tidal volume as the product of the two is minute ventilation. Initial rates of 8 to 10 breaths per minute (bpm) with a prolonged expiration time are recommended in asthma (i.e., I/E of 1:3–1:5) to allow time for full expiration and alveolar decompression.

Minute ventilation of about 10 L/min approximates a Pco$_2$ of 40 mmHg in an 80-kg adult. Minute ventilation greater then 12.5 L/min leads to hyperinflation, breath stacking, and an increased risk of baro/volutrauma. It is acceptable to permit the maintenance or gradual development of hypercapnia through reduced minute ventilation in the asthmatic patient, as this reduces peak inspiratory pressure and thus minimizes the potential for barotrauma. High intrathoracic pressure may compromise cardiac output and produce hypotension; therefore it is to be avoided.

The speed at which a mechanical breath is delivered in liters per minute, typically 60 L/min, is called the inspiratory flow (IF) rate. In asthma the initial IF should be increased to 80 to 100 L/min with a decelerating flow pattern, to allow time for the imperative prolonged expiratory phase to reduce auto-PEEP or breath stacking.

The highest measured pressure at peak inspiration is the peak inspiratory pressure (PIP). The patient's lungs, chest wall, endotracheal tube, ventilatory circuit, ventilator, and mucous plugs all contribute to the PIP. This reading has an inconsistent predictive value for baro/volutrauma but ideally should be kept under 50 cm H$_2$O. A sudden rise in PIP should be interpreted as indicating tube blockage, mucus plugging, or pneumothorax until proven otherwise. A sudden, dramatic fall in PIP may indicate extubation.

The measured intraalveolar pressure during a 0.4-second end-inspiratory pause is referred to as the plateau pressure (P$_{plat}$). Values less than 30 cm H$_2$O are best and are not usually associated with baro/volutrauma. Measurement and trending of P$_{plat}$ is an excellent objective tool to confirm optimal ventilator settings and the patient's response as well as the reversal of airflow obstruction. If initial ventilator settings disclose a P$_{plat}$ of more than 30 cm H$_2$O, consider lowering minute ventilation and increasing inspiratory flow, both of which will prolong expiratory time and attenuate hyperinflation. If P$_{plat}$ is unavailable, PIP may be used as a surrogate.

Most status asthmaticus patients who require intubation already have developed hypercapnia. The concept of controlled hypoventilation (permissive hypercapnia) promotes *gradual* development (over 3 to 4 hours) and maintenance of hypercapnia (Pco$_2$ up to 90 mmHg) and acidemia (pH as low as 7.2). This is done primarily to decrease the risk of ventilator-related lung injury and prevent hemodynamic compromise as a result of increasing intrathoracic pressure from auto-PEEP or intrinsic PEEP (PEEP$_i$). Permissive hypercapnia is usually accomplished by reducing minute ventilation, increasing inspiratory flow rate to 80 to 120 L/min, and paralyzing and heavily sedating patients who otherwise would not tolerate these settings. Permissive hypercapnia may be instrumental in promoting prolonged expiratory times and reducing auto-PEEP.

B. **Summary for initial ventilator settings**
   1. Determine the patient's ideal body weight.
   2. Set a tidal volume of 6 to 8 ml/kg.
   3. Set a respiratory rate of 8 to 10 bpm.
   4. Set an inspiratory to expiratory ratio of 1:4 to 1:5 by selecting a high inspiratory flow rate (80 to 100 L/min)
   5. Measure and maintain the plateau pressure at less than 30 cm H_2O; try to keep PIP at less than 50 cm H_2O.
   6. If necessary, allow maintenance or gradual development of hypercapnia to avoid high plateau pressures and increasing auto-PEEP.
   7. Assure continuous sedation with a benzodiazepine and paralysis with a nondepolarizing muscle relaxant.
   8. Continue in-line beta$_2$-agonist therapy and additional pharmacologic adjunctive treatment based on the severity of the patient's illness and objective response to treatment.

C. **Complications of mechanical ventilation**

Two of the more common complications seen in mechanically ventilated asthmatic patients are lung injury (baro/volutrauma) and hypotension. Lung injury is exemplified by tension pneumothorax. In those patients without tension pneumothorax, hypotension is usually related to either absolute volume depletion or relative hypovolemia caused by decreased venous return from increasing auto-PEEP and intrathoracic pressure. The inherent risks of developing either one of these complications are directly related to the degree of pulmonary hyperinflation. Of the two, hypotension occurs much more frequently than tension pneumothorax. Most asthmatic patients will be intravascularly volume depleted because of the increased work of breathing, decreased oral intake following the onset of asthmatic exacerbation, and generalized increased metabolic state. It is appropriate for these reasons to infuse up to 2 L of normal saline (NS) either before the initiation of RSI or early during mechanical ventilation.

The differential diagnosis for hypotension in the mechanically ventilated patient includes tension pneumothorax, absolute or relative decreased intravascular volume, misplaced endotracheal tube, myocardial ischemia, and metabolic acidosis. A trial of hypoventilation (apnea test) may be used to distinguish tension pneumothorax from volume depletion. The patient is disconnected from the ventilator and allowed to be apneic up to 1 minute as long as adequate oxygenation is assured by pulse oximetry. In volume depletion, the mean intrathoracic pressure will fall quickly, blood pressure should begin to rise, pulse pressure will widen, and pulse rate will fall within 30 to 60 seconds. If auto-PEEP is high, reductions in tidal volume and increases in inspiratory flow and I/E times will be required to reduce auto-PEEP. If auto-PEEP is not an issue, then an empiric volume infusion of 500 ml NS should be instituted and may be repeated based on the patient's response to the additional volume. With tension pneumothoraces, cardiopulmonary stability will not correct during the apnea time. This should prompt the immediate insertion of bilateral chest tubes and reevaluation of the patient. Obviously, lower ventilatory pressure settings will be required thereafter.

II. **Chronic obstructive pulmonary disease**

In the patient with chronic obstructive pulmonary disease (COPD), anticholinergic therapy may be as important as beta$_2$-agonist therapy. Steroids again are important to attenuate underlying inflammation. Noninvasive ventilation (BL-PAP) may be valuable in the COPD patient and may help avoid intubation. By the time COPD patients have tired and require intubation, they have usually exhausted their catecholamine stores, are usually more hypoxic than one suspects clinically, and like the asthmatic, can present significant clinical challenges once intubated. There have been recent reports in the literature of patients requiring RSI who very shortly after intubation have become bradycardic, asystolic, and were unable to be resuscitated. The physiologic explanation is not apparent. It is proposed that these patients are profoundly hypoxic before intubation, are volume depleted due to their work of breathing and their asthenic body habitus, and after intubation experience a relative sympathectomy. This vasodilates them globally, contributing to a decrease in cardiac output, which eventually results in cardiac arrest. As in the asthmatic patient, it is recommended that empiric incremental infusions of 500 ml of normal saline to a maximum of 1 to 2 L be started as soon as intubation is contemplated and that atropine and catecholamine infusions be available before intubation. These case reports, while concerning, do not reflect experience with the many COPD patients who are intubated annually.

The initial ventilator settings and potential ventilator complications discussed in the asthma patient are shared by the COPD patient.

ADDITIONAL READING

Corbridge TC, Hall JB. Techniques for ventilating patients with obstructive pulmonary disease. *J Crit Illness* 1994;9:1027–1032.

Jagoda A, Shepherd SM, Spevitz A, et al. Refractory asthma, Part I: epidemiology, pathophysiology, pharmacologic interventions. *Ann Emerg Med* 1997;29:262–274.

Kardon E. Acute asthma. *Emerg Med Clin North Am* 1996;14:93–114.

Miller RD. Nonbarbiturate intravenous anesthetics. In: Miller RD, ed. *Anesthesia,* ed. New York: Churchill Livingstone, 1994:247–289.

Strube PJ, Hallam PL. Ketamine by continuous infusion in status asthmaticus. *Anaesthesia* 1986;41:1017–1019.

Tuxen D. Permissive hypercapnic ventilation. *Am J Respir Crit Care Med* 1994;150:870–874.

21

The Distorted Airway and Upper Airway Obstruction

Michael F. Murphy

Departments of Emergency Medicine and Anaesthesiology, Queen Elizabeth II
Health Sciences Centre, Dalhousie University, Halifax, Nova Scotia

I. The clinical challenge

The anatomically difficult and disrupted airway was addressed in Chapter 5. However, the issue of upper-airway obstruction warrants specific and expanded discussion for the following reasons:

- It is important to suspect upper-airway difficulty before active airway intervention is under way, as paralysis of a patient without appreciation of airway difficulty and formulation of an appropriate plan may lead to disaster.
- The signs of upper-airway distortion and obstruction may be occult or subtle.
- The most advisable initial airway management strategy may be a cricothyrotomy.
- A predetermined protocol is advisable. The protocol should address specifically the skills, the equipment (especially special equipment such as rigid bronchoscopes), the venue, and the people that need to be involved. The fact that this airway emergency happens rarely emphasizes the importance of preplanning and practice.

The goal in these patients is to proceed rapidly in a sensible, controlled manner to manage the airway.

Anatomically, the term *upper airway* refers to that portion of the anatomy that extends from the lips and nares to the first tracheal ring. Thus the first portion of the upper airway has redundancy: a nasal path and an oral path. However, at the level of the oropharynx the two become one and the safety feature of the redundancy is lost. The most common, life-threatening causes of upper-airway distortion and obstruction occur in this common channel and are mostly laryngeal:

A. Infectious

1. Epiglottitis (also known as supraglottitis)
2. Viral and bacterial laryngotracheobronchitis (e.g., croup)
3. Parapharyngeal abscesses
4. Lingular tonsillitis (a lingual tonsil is a rare but real congenital anomaly and a well-recognized cause of failed intubation)
5. Infections or abscess of the tongue of floor or the mouth

B. Neoplastic

1. Laryngeal carcinomas
2. Hypopharyngeal and lingular (tongue) carcinomas

C. Physical and chemical agents
   1. Foreign bodies
   2. Heat/cold
   3. Acids and alkalis
   4. Inhaled toxins
D. Allergic/idiopathic, including Angiotensin Converting Enzyme Inhibitors (ACEI) angioedema
E. Traumatic: blunt and penetrating neck and upper-airway trauma

The history is extremely important and should raise the possibility of upper-airway obstruction. The best examples are burn injury to the airway and acute epiglottitis. The patient with impending upper airway obstruction is slightly hoarse or has a "hot potato" voice, resists lying flat, extends the head on the neck and juts the jaw forward, and cannot swallow secretions. These signs are often present in other causes of upper-airway obstruction. However, they may be much more subtle, and emphasis should be placed on the patient's history and presumed risk of upper-airway obstruction.

If the patient is at risk for upper-airway obstruction (e.g., stab wound to the neck), any ancillary studies such as x-rays to confirm the diagnosis must be completed promptly and using portable technique. More often than not, however, a decision needs to be made:

- Is orotracheal intubation possible?
- If so, should rapid sequence intubation (RSI) be used?
- Should the neck be prepared (prepped and local anesthetic agent infiltrated) for a surgical airway before oral intubation is attempted ("double set-up")?
- Should one proceed with an urgent surgical airway under local anesthesia?
- Is an awake laryngoscopy indicated?
- Would the intubation be better if undertaken in the operating room?

Most causes of upper-airway obstruction are associated with friable tissues and the risk of edema and bleeding with even gentle instrumentation. Due diligence and a gentle technique are required to assess the likelihood of a successful intubation. Small amounts of swelling or blood, especially in a patient who already cannot handle secretions may precipitate total obstruction and a frenzied surgical airway attempt.

II. Approach to airway management
   A. Identify the subtle signs of upper-airway obstruction. Incorporate history, patient complaints, voice character, distress, stridor, oxygen saturation, and rate of progression of symptoms and signs.
   B. Assemble the equipment and expertise required to manage the airway urgently or emergently. Have appropriately sized endotracheal tubes armed with stylets at the ready. Include the smallest cuffed endotracheal tube (ETT) available (usually 6.0 mm internal diameter). Someone capable of performing a surgical airway should be with the patient at all times, and the patient should be maintained in a resuscitation-capable area.
   C. Decide on the pace and modalities of the work-up. Is there time to do a portable soft-tissue cross-table lateral x-ray of the neck? Is fiberoptic visualization of the upper airway possible or practical?
   D. If the pace of deterioration is determined to be significant, intervene earlier rather than later.
   E. What is the risk of sedation, topical anesthesia, and a gentle look? In most instances this is possible. If the tip of the epiglottis is visible and is in the midline, orotracheal

intubation is probably possible, unless the working diagnosis is a primary laryngeal disorder, in which case more complete visualization of the larynx is mandatory (e.g., fiberoptic visualization). In these cases, direct laryngoscopy in an awake, struggling patient is ill advised.

F. If one is extremely confident that orotracheal intubation is possible, then proceed with RSI (e.g., early in the course of a penetrating neck injury). A double setup with readiness for a surgical airway is advisable. Often RSI is not considered advisable, and a controlled, urgent surgical airway is appropriate, especially if patient cooperation and time are not plentiful. Awake oral intubation with sedation and topical anesthesia may be attempted, though the risk of rapid deterioration is significant and surgical airway intervention must be swift ("double setup").

G. Percutaneous Transtracheal Ventilation (PTV) is not an option in the patient with near total upper-airway obstruction because of the inability of expired gas to find a route of exit. Nasotracheal intubation is contraindicated by the distorted anatomy.

H. Combitube or laryngeal mask airway (LMA) are options as rescue devices, though blind insertion may exacerbate the airway distortion or provoke hemorrhage.

III. Tips and pearls

A. Explore "Heliox" in your institution. Helium is less dense than nitrogen, reducing turbulent flow and resistance through tight orifices, as is the case with some causes of upper-airway obstruction. The commercial preparations are usually 80% helium and 20% oxygen, and provided lung function is adequate, this mix will produce acceptable oxygen saturations. This may buy time if required.

B. Get familiar with a fiberoptic scope and use it regularly to do diagnostic work so you are familiar with the procedure and the anatomy of the upper airway.

C. Have clear protocols and algorithms in place for this emergency.

D. Zone II and lower zone III penetrating neck injuries are best managed nonsurgically or may require tracheostomy, not cricothyrotomy. This is all the more reason for early RSI before anatomic distortion occurs. All gunshot wounds of the neck should be intubated before there is any sign of hematoma or distortion. In general, if there is evidence of direct airway injury (subcutaneous air) or vascular injury (bleeding or hematoma), then early active airway management is indicated.

E. Crush injuries to the larynx and laryngeal fractures are best managed with tracheostomy rather than cricothyrotomy, or RSI circumstances permitting.

F. In the event of a tracheal separation (e.g. clothesline-type injury to the neck) when one is performing a surgical airway, grasp the distal stump before opening the pretracheal fascia.

G. The patient with a bulky pharyngeal or laryngeal tumor may be intubated using a fiberoptic technique, and this is preferable to invading an airway that may be subject to a later operative resection.

ADDITIONAL READING

Barratt GE, Coulthard SW. Upper airway obstruction: diagnosis and management. In: Brown BR, ed. *Contemporary anaesthesia practice.* Philadelphia: FA Davis, 1987.

Dougherty TB. The difficult airway in conventional head and neck surgery. In: Benumof JL, ed. *Airway management: principles and practice.* St Louis: Mosby, 1996.

Heindel DJ. Deep neck abscesses in the adult: management of a difficult airway. *Anesth Analg* 1987;66:774.

Walls RM, Wolfe R, Rosen P. Fools rush in? Airway management in penetrating neck trauma. Editorial. *J Emerg Med* 1993;11:479–480.

22

The Critically Ill Patient

Michael F. Murphy

*Departments of Emergency Medicine and Anaesthesiology, Queen Elizabeth II
Health Sciences Centre, Dalhousie University, Halifax, Nova Scotia*

Patients with limited cardiopulmonary reserve or even frank cardiopulmonary failure present a complex challenge when it comes to endotracheal intubation. On the one hand, one is reluctant to administer medications that may further compromise physiologic status. On the other hand, endotracheal intubation is associated with substantial reflex responses that have the potential to lead to further cardiovascular decompensation. Balancing these is difficult.

Appropriate decision making and actions depend on a detailed understanding of the organ system responses to intubation, the effects of pharmacologic agents to be used to facilitate intubation, and the balance to be sought in each individual patient. This is a crucial decision in the patient who is critically ill, as small variations in technique or drug doses may have significant consequences.

I. **Organ system responses to endotracheal intubation**
   The larynx is the most heavily innervated sensory structure in the body:
   - The glossopharyngeal nerve supplies the pharynx and hypopharynx, including pharyngeal (anterior) surface of epiglottis
   - The vagus nerve supplies the larynx:
      Superior laryngeal branches: laryngeal (posterior) surface of the epiglottis and the remainder of the larynx above the level of vocal cords
      Recurrent laryngeal nerves: sensory supply to the larynx and trachea below the level of the vocal cords

   Because of this intense sensory supply, stimulation results in aggressive physiologic responses that, if unchecked, have the potential to produce significant, adverse end organ consequences. In the critically ill patient the following organ system responses are the most important to consider:
   A. **The upper airway and respiratory system**
      - Glottic closure or "laryngospasm" (combined adduction of false and true cords)
      - Increased oropharyngeal, tracheal, and bronchial secretions
      - Bronchoconstriction
      - Stimulation of the "gag reflex"
      - Coughing and "bucking"
   B. **The autonomic nervous system**
      1. Adrenergic responses
         - Increased sympathetic and adrenal response with elevated circulating catecholamines:

Increased systolic blood pressure (SBP) and mean arterial blood pressure (MAP) (up to two times normal); increased diastolic blood pressure (DBP) (up to 50% increase);

Increased heart rate (HR) (up to 50% increase); increased cardiac work and myocardial oxygen consumption (MVO_2)

Ventricular dysrhythmias (increased automaticity/irritability due to increased circulating catecholamines and increased blood pressure)

Decreased gastric emptying (increased gastric volume and risk of aspiration) and decreased gut motility (ileus)

2. Cholinergic responses:
   - Bronchoconstriction and bronchorrhea
   - Bradycardia: rarely but occasionally in children and infants, especially if hypoxemic

Laryngoscopy and endotracheal intubation summate to produce these physiologic effects. The intensity of the physiologic responses is related to the intensity of stimulation, which depends upon

- The duration of laryngoscopy
- The aggressiveness of laryngoscopy
- The degree of attendant hypoxemia/hypercarbia
- Stimulation of the carina by the endotracheal tube
- The use of alternative placement techniques (e.g., lightwand) that produce less stimulation
- The use of a nontracheal device (e.g., laryngeal mask airway), inducing less stimulation

II. Patients at risk

All patients should be considered as potentially at risk from the adverse cardiovascular and pulmonary responses to endotracheal intubation. However, those already critically ill are especially so. Underlying conditions of particular note include the following:

A. The upper airway and respiratory system
- Reactive airways disease

B. The cardiovascular system
- Ischemic heart disease (IHD)
- Left ventricular dysfunction ("failure") due to any etiology:
  Ischemic
  Hypertensive heart disease
  Cardiomyopathies
- Valvular heart disease
- Congenital heart disease:
  L to R shunts (e.g., ventricular septal defect (VSD))
- Cor pulmonale
- Ventricular and atrial arrhythmias may be induced
- Aortic dissection and rupture
- Major vessel aneurysm rupture (congenital, traumatic, or atherosclerotic)

C. The brain
- Patients with intracranial hypertension or increased intracranial pressure (ICP)

III. Mitigating and preventing the adverse physiologic responses to intubation

A. Nonpharmacologic methods
Increasing stimulation of the larynx proportionately increases the adrenergic and ICP responses to intubation. Thus limiting the time and forcefulness of laryngoscopy re-

duces the magnitude of adverse physiologic response. Preoxygenation (Chapter 2) limits the possibility of desaturation during intubation, avoiding the adrenergic response resulting from hypoxemia. There is also some evidence the laryngeal stimulation during intubation with a lightwand is less than that which occurs when conventional laryngoscopy is performed.

In summary, the nonpharmacologic methods of limiting the adverse physiologic responses to intubation include the following:

- Limit the time of laryngoscopy
- Preoxygenate and use a pulse oximeter
- Hyperventilate by bag and mask (decrease $PaCO_2$), especially if increased ICP or impaired autoregulation is suspected
- Use an alternative technique that is associated with less stimulation, if reasonable (e.g., lightwand or ILM)
- Pass the endotracheal tube in an atraumatic way
- Keep the tube off the carina

B. Pharmacologic methods

Every time you use a medication to attenuate the physiologic responses to intubation consider the following (see box 22.1):

1. The additive or potentiating effects of one technique or drug on another (e.g., patients with total upper-airway anesthesia may require less induction agent; intoxicated patients need less induction agent; the use of fentanyl supplements the induction agent and less induction agent may be required).

2. The patient's physiologic reserve: Patients with reduced cardiac reserve (decreased left ventrical (LV) function and valvular heart disease) are more sensitive to myocardial depressants such as induction agents, as are patients that are hypovolemic, such as those with uncontrolled hypertension, blood loss, or dehydration.

3. The potential of an adverse outcome related to the physiologic response to intubation: The physiologic response to intubation may be especially detrimental in patients with significant moderate to severe asthma, ischemic heart disease (IHD), elevated ICP, intracranial hemorrhage, and rupturing or dissecting aneurysms.

4. Underlying sympathetic tone: If the sympathetic nervous system is already maximally stimulated (e.g., hemorrhagic shock) and the patient is barely compensated, one must be cautious with any drug that can reduce sympathetic tone. This includes all sedative hypnotic agents (alcohol, benzodiazepines, barbiturates), neuroleptics (haloperidol and droperidol), opioids, lidocaine, and histamine releasers. Etomidate, ketamine, succinylcholine, and pancuronium are the safest bets. For sedation, small titrated doses of fentanyl or haloperidol are probably safer than benzodiazepines or barbiturates.

When using medications to mitigate the adverse physiologic responses to intubation in patients with marginal pulmonary or cardiovascular reserve (e.g. those that are critically ill), ad-

---

Box 22.1

Balance the need to control the response against the capacity of the patient to respond to the stimulus.

minister conservative doses and err on the side of "too little" rather than "too much." If postintubation hypertension and tachycardia occur, they can be managed by administering small doses of the induction agent or by titrating a benzodiazepine or opioid (e.g. fentanyl).

IV. Acute pulmonary edema

A. The clinical challenge

The patient with acute pulmonary edema due to left ventricular failure who requires intubation presents several challenges to the physician performing the intubation:

- Preoxygenation will provide little in the way of oxygen reserve, as these patients have little or no functional residual capacity (FRC)
- The patient may be unable to lie flat and is often struggling and uncooperative, presenting airway access difficulties
- Foamy secretions may obscure visualization of the airway
- High airway resistance and low pulmonary compliance are likely to render bag-and-mask ventilation ineffective
- Cardiac reserve varies. The patient who is hypertensive is more likely to tolerate opioids and induction agents than one who is normotensive, who in turn is more likely to tolerate opioids and induction agents than a hypotensive patient
- Intubation is likely to exacerbate any element of bronchospasm

All these points emphasize the fact that there is little margin for error in these patients and that intubation should be atraumatic, swift, and successful on the first attempt whenever possible. This argues strongly for the superior pharmacologic and physical control, and success rates provided by rapid sequence intubation (RSI)

B. Approach to airway management

1. Attempt to preoxygenate with 100% oxygen, even though it may not be as effective as in patients with normal lungs. Assist ventilation to keep oxygen saturation if at all possible.
2. Positioning: The cardiovascular system will tolerate the procedure, medications, and ventilation better in the supine position, but the patient usually prefers to be erect. It may be best to administer drugs with the patient erect and then to place the patient in a supine position for intubation.
3. Account for medications that have already been administered, noting particularly those with sympathetic or cardiovascular effects (e.g., benzodiazepines, nitrates, opioids, etc).
4. Assess cardiovascular reserve. Patients who are hypertensive and hyperdynamic have the capacity to respond aggressively to intubation and will require medications to attenuate this response. Use caution in patients who are normotensive and extreme caution in those who are hypotensive.
5. Draw up RSI drugs, including fentanyl, etomidate, succinylcholine, pancuronium, or vecuronium. Have intravenous nitroglycerine available. Pressors such as dobutamine, dopamine, or ephedrine should be available. Alpha agent pressors such as phenylephrine and methoxamine are inappropriate, as they increase blood pressure at the expense of increased left ventricular myocardial oxygen consumption. An exception is the patient with significant aortic or mitral stenosis and a fixed cardiac output, in which case alpha-adrenergic agonists may be preferable.
6. Use as large an endotracheal tube as you will be able to insert through the cords to minimize resistance to ventilation and facilitate pulmonary toilette (8 to 9 mm ID in an adult female; 9 to 10 mm ID in an adult male). Place a stylet in the tube.
7. Assess the airway. If the airway appears difficult and you are not confident that the intubation will be swift, atraumatic, and successful, an awake intubation is

advisable. Note, however, that awake intubation will be more stimulating and carries a higher complication and failure rate than RSI.

C. Recommended intubation sequence

Leave the patient upright with the head of the bed elevated:

1. Preparation
2. Preoxygenation
3. Pretreatment
   a. fentanyl 3 μ/kg intravenously (IV) if the patient is hypertensive; reduced to 1 to 1.5 μ/kg if normotensive; avoid altogether if hypotensive.
4. Paralysis with induction
   a. Etomidate 0.3 mg/kg if hypertensive or normotensive; reduce to 0.2 mg/kg if hypotensive
   b. Succinylcholine 1.5 mg/kg
5. Protection and positioning
   a. Sellick's maneuver
   b. Place patient supine
6. Placement with proof
   a. gentle intubation
7. Postintubation management
   a. Confirm tube placement with End tidal Carbon dioxide ($ETCO_2$)
   b. Titrate diazepam to ensure the patient is sedated (0.1 to 0.2 mg/kg IV to start)
   c. Administer 0.1 mg/kg pancuronium or vecuronium to facilitate mechanical ventilation

D. Initiating mechanical ventilation

1. Immediately after intubation, bag-ventilate the patient to get some idea of compliance and resistance. Appreciate the time needed to complete expiration. Note the volume of secretions. Get the oxygen saturations into the 90+ range if possible. Note the effect of positive pressure ventilation on blood pressure. Obtain a chest x-ray and look especially carefully for a right mainstem intubation, as one lung ventilation is even less tolerated when the patient has pulmonary edema.
2. Set the F_iO_2 at 100%. A tidal of 10 ml/kg at a rate of 10 breaths/min, as usual, is a good place to start.
3. An elevated mean intrathoracic pressure due to positive pressure ventilation may impede venous return and improve left ventricular function in the setting of acute left ventricular failure, though peak airway pressures exceeding 35 to 40 cm of water pressure (CWP) are associated with an increased risk of pneumothorax. Increased intrathoracic pressure must be traded off against a compromise of cardiac output.
4. In the event that the lungs are very stiff and high airway pressures are compromising venous return and cardiac output, faster rates at lower tidal volumes may be required.
5. If there is significant bronchospasm, the rate may have to be decreased to extend the expiratory time and the tidal volume increased, if possible, to maintain minute volume.
6. Once the rate and volume are reasonable, Positive End Expiratory Pressure (PEEP) beginning at 5 Centimeters Water Pressure (CWP) or other forms of pressure support may be introduced to enhance FRC and oxygenation if the cardiac output will tolerate it. Increase the PEEP as needed and as tolerated.
7. Treat the pulmonary edema aggressively according to its cause.

E. **Tips and pearls**
  1. Dramatic falls in blood pressure with drugs (especially nitrates and histamine releasers) and ventilation may tip you off to underlying significant valvular heart disease.
  2. In the patient with hypertension immediately after intubation, small repeated doses of thiopentone (25 to 50 mg) or propofol (10 to 20 mg) may be used to both sedate and lower the blood pressure. However, postintubation hypertension that persists is the result of inadequate sedation and excessive sympathetic tone. Diazepam, supplemented with morphine or fentanyl, and nitrates constitute a good approach.
  3. Circulation times are slowed in these patients and medication onset time may be considerably delayed.

V. **Cardiogenic shock**
  A. **The clinical challenge**
    The patient in cardiogenic shock is gravely ill and likely to die. This fact serves to emphasize the attention to detail that is required in managing the intubation.
    • Provided the patient is not in heart failure, the FRC is probably intact and preoxygenation is useful
    • By definition, there is no cardiac reserve, and any medication used to facilitate intubation that reduces cardiovascular performance is contraindicated
    • The challenge is to determine if a small dose of an amnestic agent such as midazolam 0.5 to 1 mg is indicated in the awake and alert patient prior to intubation Etomidate and ketamine should be avoided, as both can depress cardiac function
    • Long-term sedation with diazepam in small titrated doses of 1 to 2 mg may be tolerated
    • Circulation times are prolonged, so drug effects are substantially delayed
  B. **Approach to airway management**
    • Evaluate the airway
    • As with the patient in pulmonary edema, there is little margin for error in this patient and intubation should be atraumatic, swift, and successful on the first attempt
    • Be prepared to handle surges in blood pressure and myocardial oxygen demand after intubation, rather than preemptively
    1. Recommended sequence:
      a. Preparation
      b. Preoxygenation
      c. Pretreatment
        • None
      d. Paralysis with induction
        • No induction agent; perhaps 0.5 to 1 mg of midazolam as an amnestic agent.
        • Succinylcholine 1.5 mg/kg
      e. Protection and positioning
        • Sellick's maneuver
        • Position patient for intubation
      f. Placement with proof
        • gentle, atraumatic intubation
      g. Postintubation management
        • Diazepam 1 to 2 mg increments
        • Pancuronium 0.1 mg/kg

C. Initiating mechanical ventilation
- Be cautious of impeding venous return and cardiac filling with vigorous ventilation

D. Tips and pearls

Paralytic agents such as succinylcholine do not have substantial cardiovascular activity. Pancuronium has sympathomimetic activity, though it is unlikely to be evident in the setting of cardiogenic shock, where sympathetic activity is already maximal. Histamine-releasing agents such as the benzylisoquinoline neuromuscular blocking agents (NMBAs) ought to be avoided.

VI. Septic shock

A. The clinical challenge
1. Septic shock may be hyperdynamic or hypodynamic; myocardial contractility and systemic vascular resistance are compromised. The challenge is to maintain cardiac output and oxygen delivery to the tissues.
2. Any agent that may compromise myocardial contractility or systemic vascular resistance is contraindicated.

B. Approach to airway management
1. Evaluate the airway.
2. The approach to airway management in the patient with septic shock is no different from that in the patient in cardiogenic shock (see recommended sequence earlier).

C. Initiating mechanical ventilation
1. Ventilation should be initiated at 10 ml/kg at 10 breaths/min. However, as most patients in septic shock are also acidemic, consideration should be given to increasing minute ventilation by 20% to 30%, if the cardiac output will tolerate it, until arterial blood gasses (ABGs) can be obtained.
2. Pressure support may reduce shunt fraction and improve oxygenation, provided cardiac output is maintained.

D. Tips and pearls
1. Be cautious with ventilation. Any reduction in venous return will not be tolerated.
2. Be meticulous in ensuring an endobronchial intubation is avoided.

VII. Anaphylaxis

A. The clinical challenge
1. The patient suffering from a systemic anaphylactic reaction demonstrates hypotension due to profound histamine-induced vasodilatation, intense bronchoconstriction, and upper-airway edema.
2. The patient may be profoundly acidemic (respiratory and metabolic).
3. Orotracheal intubation with a large-bore endotracheal tube that minimizes resistance and permits aggressive bronchial toilette is desirable.
4. Orotracheal intubation is potentially complicated by upper-airway edema, and emergency surgical airway intervention may be necessary. PTV and other rescue airway devices such as Combitubes and laryngeal mask airways will be ineffective because of the combination of upper-airway obstruction and bronchospasm.
5. Hypotension limits the spectrum of pharmacologic options for sedation.
6. Intense bronchospasm will challenge the ability to ventilate the patient effectively and attenuate the mixed acidosis that is present.

B. Approach to airway management
1. There is little margin for error in this patient, and intubation should be atraumatic, swift, and successful on the first attempt.

Box 22.2

Time	Action
Zero minus 10 minutes	Preparation
Zero minus 5 minutes	Preoxygenation
Zero minus 3 minutes	Pretreatment: lidocaine 1.0 mg/kg
Zero	Paralysis with induction:ketamine 1.5 mg/kg; succinylcholine 1.5 mg/kg
	Protection and positioning
Zero plus 20 to 30 seconds	
Zero plus 45 seconds	Placement with proof: Perform intubation
	Postintubation management
Zero plus 60 seconds	Confirm tube placement
	Continue to treat anaphylaxis

---

2. Intense bronchospasm and hypotension will limit the effectiveness of preoxygenation and gas exchange in the preintubation period. Therefore expeditious intubation is desired.
3. Prepare to perform a surgical airway.
4. If you are confident in your ability to intubate the patient, maximize the success rate by using RSI. If upper-airway edema or stridor is present, an awake technique or primary cricothyrotomy is recommended.
5. Treat the anaphylaxis, especially with epinephrine, during preparation for intubation.
6. Ketamine provides the best blood pressure support and is a bronchodilator.

C. **Recommended Sequence (Box 22.2)**
D. **Initiating mechanical ventilation**
   1. The substantial increase in airways resistance will mandate slow rates and moderate tidal volumes with permissive hypercapnia in order to achieve acceptable oxygenation and minimal barotrauma.
   2. Excessive mean intrathoracic pressure is likely to compromise venous return and cardiac output.

E. **Tips and pearls**
   • Avoid pure alpha-adrenergic agents to manage hypotension, as there is the theoretical potential of augmenting bronchospasm.
   • Pancuronium is the relaxant of choice. Benzylisoquinoline derivatives (e.g., curare, cis-atracurium) are to be avoided because of their ability to release histamine.

ADDITIONAL READING

Bishop MJ, Bedford RF, Kil HK. Physiologic and pathophysiologic responses to intubation. In: Benumof JL, ed. *Airway management: principles and practice.* St Louis: Mosby, 1996.

Fox EJ, Sklar GS, Hill CH, et al: Complications related to the pressor response to endotracheal intubation. *Anaesthesiology* 1977;47:524–525.

Habib MP. Physiologic implications of artificial airways. *Chest* 1989;96:180.

23

The Pregnant Patient

Michael F. Murphy

Departments of Emergency Medicine and Anaesthesiology,
Queen Elizabeth II Health Sciences Centre, Dalhousie University, Halifax, Nova Scotia

I. The clinical challenge

Complications related to airway management represent the most significant cause of anesthetic-related maternal mortality. However, pregnant patients who present to the emergency department are more likely to die from their illness or injury than an airway management misadventure. The point, however, should not be lost because it emphasizes the importance of emergency airway management skills in pregnant patients.

Airway management in the pregnant patient must take into account the stage of the pregnancy as well as anatomic and pathophysiologic conditions that antedate the pregnancy.

The unique features of the pregnant patient to be considered in airway management, especially in the last trimester and particularly near term, include the following:

1. Difficult intubation is more common in the pregnant patient at or near term due to several contributing factors:
   - Weight gain during pregnancy
   - Larger breasts, which may obstruct access to the anterior neck for Sellick's maneuver or a surgical airway
   - Upper-airway edema and mucosal congestion (especially in toxemia)
2. A reduced functional residual capacity (FRC) and increased rate of oxygen consumption results in more rapid desaturation if apneic.
3. Increased risk of regurgitation and aspiration of gastric contents caused by
   - Increased gastric volume and lower pH
   - Delayed gastric emptying
   - Increased incidence of gastroesophageal reflux (increased intraabdominal pressure, reduced lower esophageal sphincter tone)
4. Vena caval compression in the supine position results in decreased venous return and cardiac output in the last trimester. The administration of induction agents may substantially reduce cardiac output and placental perfusion.
5. Peripheral and pulmonary vascular resistance are decreased throughout pregnancy; blood pressure is decreased and pulse pressure is increased.
6. Bag-and-mask ventilation may be more difficult because of the weight of the breasts on the chest wall and the increase in intraabdominal pressure caused by the gravid uterus, restricting diaphragmatic excursion.

With each maneuver or intervention, placental perfusion and oxygen delivery to the fetus must be considered. As a general rule, "What's good for the mother is good for the fetus."

II. Approach to airway management

The sequence of events in managing the airway of the pregnant patient is no different from that of any other intubation in the emergency department, except for the unique features of pregnancy as described earlier:

1. Assemble rescue airway equipment and be prepared for the difficult airway. Remember that the mucosa may be engorged, edematous, and friable. Nasotracheal intubation is more likely to lead to mucosal damage and bleeding.
2. Preoxygenate, remembering that the FRC is reduced, oxygen consumption is increased, and apnea leads to desaturation more rapidly.
3. Attenuating the autonomic and cardiovascular responses to intubation with opioids and induction agents may lead to a reduction in maternal cardiac output and placental perfusion and must be weighed carefully in the context of the clinical situation. In addition, opioids and induction agents cross the placental barrier and may depress the neonate in the event that delivery is imminent. Muscle relaxants do not cross the placenta. In general, keep the intubation sequence as simple as possible.
4. An assistant trained in the application of cricoid pressure is essential in this situation. Cricoid pressure must be uninterrupted until the airway is secured, as always, but particular attention is important here.
5. While rescue airway devices such as the Intubating Laryngeal Mask (ILM) and the Combitube fill a similar role in the event that intubation fails, the enhanced risk of aspiration must be appreciated and definitive airway control expedited.

III. Recommended intubation sequence

A. Preparation
B. Preoxygenation
1. 100% oxygen
2. Tilt the abdomen slightly to the left with a wedge or pillow under the right hip to displace the gravid uterus from the inferior vena cava (IVC) and prevent the "supine hypotensive syndrome" of pregnancy.

C. Pretreatment
1. Avoid pretreatment drugs unless they are truly indicated.

D. Paralysis with induction
1. Etomidate 0.3 mg/kg
2. Succinylcholine 1.5 mg/kg

E. Protection and positioning
1. Sellick's maneuver

F. Placement with proof
1. Be gentle; the tissues may be friable

G. Postintubation management
1. See later with respect to mechanical ventilation.
2. Ensure tracheal placement of the tube with a carbon dioxide detection device *before* releasing Sellick's maneuver.

IV. Initiating mechanical ventilation

Pregnancy is associated with an increased metabolic rate, with the need to increase minute ventilation as the pregnancy progresses. At term, this translates into a 30% to 50% increase in minute ventilation. Arterial blood gases or pulse oximetry and end-tidal carbon dioxide monitoring will aid in adjusting the ventilation parameters. Modest adjustments of both rate (start at 12/minute) and tidal volume (start at 12 cc/kg) will meet the ventilatory need.

V. Tips and pearls

In the third trimester a substantial proportion of pregnant patients will suffer from the "supine hypotensive syndrome" if placed in the supine position. Vena caval compression is likely the cause, and substantial reductions in placental perfusion may result, with attendant fetal distress. All pregnant patients in the last trimester, especially those near term, should have their abdomen tilted to the left by elevating the right hip with a pillow or intravenous bag.

Pregnant patients are hard to ventilate with a bag and mask. Be prepared to use a two-handed technique and achieve a definitive airway (endotracheal intubation) as rapidly as possible.

ADDITIONAL READING

Crosby ET. The difficult airway in obstetric anaesthesia. In: Benumof JL, ed. *Airway management: principles and practice.* St Louis: Mosby, 1996.

24

Prolonged Seizure Activity

Robert J. Vissers

*Department of Emergency Medicine, University of North Carolina,
Chapel Hill, North Carolina*

I. The clinical challenge

A general discussion of the diagnosis and treatment of seizure disorder is beyond the scope of this book. This chapter will focus primarily on the considerations of airway management in the seizure patient. In the simple, self-limited, grand mal seizure, airway management is directed at termination of the seizure and prevention of hypoxia from airway obstruction. Paralysis and intubation should be considered when SpO_2 falls below 90% or when typical first-line measures fail to terminate the seizure in a reasonable time period. For the simple seizure, basic airway maneuvers, expectant observation (most seizures end spontaneously), supplemental high-flow oxygen, and vigilance are usually all that is necessary. Airway protection from aspiration is rarely required in the simple, self-limited seizure because the uncoordinated motor activity precludes coordinated expulsion of gastric contents.

Determining when to proceed from supportive measures to intubation is one of the clinical challenges in the airway management of the seizing patient. Status epilepticus is defined as continuous seizure activity for 30 minutes or multiple seizures without recovery of consciousness in between. Although useful in discussions of seizure management, status epilepticus is less precise with regard to indications for airway management. Therefore the discussion will focus on when intubation may be indicated in the patient with prolonged seizure activity. The absolute and relative indications for intubation in the seizing patient are listed in Box 24.1.

II. Approach to airway management in the seizing patient

A. Self-limited seizure

Most seizures terminate rapidly, either spontaneously or in response to medication, and require only supportive measures. Positioning the patient on his or her side, providing oxygen by face mask, suctioning secretions and blood carefully, and occasionally using the jaw thrust to relieve obstruction from the tongue are usually all that is necessary to prevent hypoxia and aspiration. It is often impossible to introduce a bite block or oral airway in the seizing patient, and such attempts may cause dental trauma. Attempts to ventilate during a seizure are usually ineffective and rarely necessary.

B. Prolonged seizure activity

Although most self-limited seizures do not require intubation, there are several indications for intubation in the prolonged seizure. Extensive generalized motor activity will

---

Box 24.1.   Indications for endotracheal intubation

Absolute indications
1. Hypoxemia (SpO_2 < 90%) secondary to hypoventilation or airway obstruction
2. Treatment of underlying etiology (e.g., intracranial bleed with elevated intracranial pressure)
3. Cessation of a prolonged seizure refractory to anticonvulsants to prevent accumulating metabolic debt (acidosis, rhabdomyolysis)
4. Generalized status epilepticus

Relative indications
1. Prophylaxis for the respiratory depressant effect of anticonvulsants (e.g., benzodiazepines, barbiturates)
2. Termination of seizure activity to facilitate diagnostic workup (e.g., computed tomography scanning)
3. Airway protection in prolonged seizures.

---

eventually cause hypoxia, significant acidosis, rhabdomyolysis, and hyperthermia. Respiratory depression may result from high doses or combinations of anticonvulsants. Oxygen saturation of less than 90%, despite supplemental, high-flow oxygen, is an indication for immediate intubation.

There is no clear guideline that specifically defines the duration of seizure activity requiring intubation. A good rule of thumb is that seizures lasting more than 10 minutes despite appropriate anticonvulsant therapy should be considered for intubation. Generally, when first-line (benzodiazepine) anticonvulsants fail to terminate grand mal seizure activity, rapid sequence intubation (RSI) is indicated. Phosphenytoin, which has a relatively short loading time, may be initiated as a second-line agent before intubation, if time allows. Other second-line anticonvulsants (phenytoin, phenobarbital) require at least 20 more minutes for a loading dose; therefore at the time of initiation of such a load, intubation is advisable.

C. Technique of intubation

RSI is the method of choice in the seizing patient. In addition to its technical superiority, RSI ends all motor activity, allowing the body to begin to correct the metabolic debt. However, cessation of motor activity while the patient is paralyzed does not represent termination of the seizure, and fully effective loading doses of appropriate anticonvulsants (e.g., phenytoin) are required immediately after intubation. The recommended technique for the seizure patient is described in box 24.2.

Standard RSI technique is appropriate in the seizing patient with the following modifications:

1. Preoxygenation may be suboptimal because of uncoordinated respiratory effort; therefore pulse oximetry is critical.

2. Sodium pentothal shares anticonvulsant activity with its barbiturate siblings and may be the best choice for induction in the absence of hypotension (Chapter 15). Midazolam is an appropriate alternative. Etomidate has an unclear effect on seizure activity and therefore should be considered only if associated hypotension precludes the

---

Box 24.2

Time	Action	
Zero minus 10 minutes	Preparation	
Zero minus 5 minutes	Preoxygenation	Continue anticonvulsant Rx
Zero minus 3 minutes	Pretreatment	Continue anticonvulsant Rx
Zero	Paralysis with induction:	Sodium thiopental* 3mg/kg Succinylcholine 1.5 mg/kg
Zero plus 20 to 30 seconds	Protection and positioning	
Zero plus 45 seconds	Placement with proof:	Perform intubation
Zero plus 60 seconds	Postintubation management	Continue anticonvulsant Rx Vecoronium 0.1 mg/kg IV Diazepam 0.2 mg/kg IV

*Midazolam 0.3 mg/kg may be substituted.

---

use of pentothal or midazolam. Although etomidate may raise the seizure threshold (and therefore inhibit seizure activity) in generalized seizures, it lowers the threshold in focal seizures. Little data exist on propofol as an induction agent in patients with seizures; however, EEG activity may actually be increased in lower doses.

3. Prolonged paralysis with pancuronium or vecuronium and sedation with an additional benzodiazepine is desirable for the first hour after intubation to facilitate investigations (e.g., CT scan) and to allow acidosis to correct with controlled ventilation.

4. Continuous bedside EEG monitoring is necessary in the paralyzed patient to assess for ongoing seizure activity. If this is not immediately available, motor paralysis should frequently be allowed to wear off to evaluate the effectiveness of anticonvulsant therapy.

5. If elevated intracanial pressure (ICP), head injury, known central nervous system pathology, or suspected meningitis is present, ICP intubation technique (Chapter 19) should be used.

D. **Pitfalls**

1. Always ensure that hypoglycemia is not the cause of the seizure. Check glucose or administer intravenous dextrose solution in all cases.

2. Nasal intubation is possible in the seizing patient but is of little use. RSI will permit faster intubation and will stop the motor activity.

3. The paralyzed patient is often still seizing. Administer effective doses of long-acting anticonvulsants and use benzodiazepines for long-term sedation. Arrange continuous electroencephalography monitoring, if possible, or allow motor recovery frequently (at least every hour) to assess response to therapy.

4. Prolonged seizure activity almost always represents a significant change in seizure pattern for the patient. A careful search for an underlying cause, including head CT scan, is indicated.

ADDITIONAL READING

Bradford JC, Kyriakedes CG. Evaluation of the patient with seizures: an evidence-based approach. *Emerg Med Clinic North Am* 1999;17:203–220.

Engel J, Starkman S. Overview of seizures. *Emerg Med Clin North Am* 1994;12:895.

Pollack CV, Pollack ES. Seizures. In: Rosen P, Barkin R, Danzl DF, et al., eds. *Emergency medicine: concepts and clinical practice,* 4th ed. St Louis: Mosby, 1998.

Willmore LJ. Epilepsy emergencies: the first seizure and status epileptics. *Neurology* 1998;51:534–538.

25

The Geriatric Patient

Diane M. Birnbaumer

Department of Emergency Medicine, Harbor-UCLA Medical Center, Torrance, California

Advanced age is characterized by a loss of physiologic reserve. Aspects of aging affect virtually every consideration in airway management from the decision to intubate to the choice and doses of pharmacologic agents.

I. The decision to intubate

Aging affects the decision to intubate in three primary areas. First, the elderly patient may not have the respiratory reserve and energy to continue breathing effectively against the resistance caused by the respiratory threat. The work of breathing in this setting can be substantially increased and can rapidly deplete the patient's muscular energy stores. The patient may already have chronic lung disease, compromising oxygenation even at baseline. Comorbidity, such as ischemic heart disease, may reduce the patient's tolerance of hypoxemia. Medications, especially antihypertensives and psychotropic medications, may further compromise the patient's ability to generate adequate respiratory effort. All these elements combine to make the elderly patient less able to sustain or overcome prolonged or severe respiratory compromise. Thus the decision to intubate may occur at an earlier point in the course of the respiratory or airway emergency. Second, elderly patients have a disproportionately increased incidence of difficult airways, primarily because of reduced mobility in the temporomandibular joint and cervical spine, caused by degenerative processes. Thus one might start planning the approach to the airway earlier than in a younger patient to permit time to assess the airway adequately and to plan for contingencies. The third, and potentially most challenging, effect of aging is on the ethical considerations regarding intubation. Many elderly patients, especially those with debilitating, chronic disease (including chronic obstructive pulmonary disease), have expressed their wish not to be intubated. When such expression is manifested on a properly executed, recently (<6 months) dated, legal advance directive, and when the patient can verbalize his or her agreement with this directive, the physician may confidently abstain from intubation. When one or more of these criteria are not met or when the patient cannot verbalize but family members state that the patient has recanted and would desire intubation, the decision making is much more complex. A full discussion of these issues is beyond the scope of this manual. In general, where information is contradictory or incomplete, the physician or provider must take such action as he or she believes the patient would want. It is widely advocated that a provider forced to choose between aggressive intervention and potentially fatal inaction in the context of incomplete information should choose the course most likely to keep the patient alive until more information is available.

II. Approach to the airway

The standard approach to airway management involves several steps. First, the patient should be assessed to determine if a potentially difficult airway exists. In the absence of a difficult airway, rapid sequence intubation (RSI) should be performed. In cases of difficult or failed airways, rescue devices may be needed. Each of these areas may be affected by the changes seen in aging.

Elderly patients may be more likely to require use of the difficult airway algorithm. Elderly patients often have dentures, which may interfere with laryngoscopy and should be removed just before laryngoscopy. However, if bagging is necessary in these edentulous patients, this lack of teeth may impede mask seal and interfere with effective ventilation, so unless dentures are obstructing the airway, they should remain in place until immediately before laryngoscopy. Temporomandibular joint arthritis that limits mouth opening will be detected when evaluating the 3-3-2 rule. This will also reduce the Mallampati score and make laryngoscopy more difficult. When evaluating for airway obstruction, elderly patients are more likely than younger patients to have a history of airway surgery or irradiation. Neck mobility may be affected by cervical spine arthritis. This can limit the ability to line up the airway axes, making intubation and visualization more problematic and at times frankly impossible.

Despite the preceding problems, most elderly patients are candidates for RSI. RSI may require modification because of the changes seen with aging.

A. Preparation

Preparation should always include easy access to suctioning and readiness to turn the patient into the lateral decubitus position, as aspiration risk and morbidity are higher in the elderly. Aging leads to decreased lower esophageal sphincter tone, which increases the risk of aspiration. If aspiration occurs, outcome is worse in the elderly patient than in a younger patient, with more severe morbidity and increased mortality.

B. Preoxygenation

Preoxygenation, a critical step for maximizing oxygen reserve during intubation, may be less effective in the elderly. Underlying heart and lung disease, and decreased reserve often limit the amount of preoxygenation achievable in these patients. Oxygen desaturation will occur more quickly in the elderly, who behave like the "moderately ill" adult in Figure 2.1. This oxygen saturation should be meticulously monitored, and bag-and-mask ventilation should be initiated if oxygen saturations fall below 90%.

C. Pretreatment

Pretreatment with fentanyl can be very important in the elderly, as it will blunt the catecholamine response to intubation, which may be detrimental in this population with a high rate of cardiovascular and cerebrovascular disease. On the other hand, fentanyl should be used cautiously, as elderly patients may be particularly sensitive to the respiratory depressant effects of opioids. Use of fentanyl in lower doses (1 to 2 μg/kg) is prudent, and the fentanyl should be given slowly, over 2 to 3 minutes.

D. Paralytic

Paralytic use should not be affected by age, and the use of paralytic agents to achieve muscle relaxation is as important in the elderly as it is in younger patients. When etomidate is used as the induction agent, no changes are necessary in the elderly. However, when midazolam is used, the dose should be reduced to one-third to one-half, as the elderly may become hypotensive with typical induction doses of 0.3 mg/kg. In general, a dose of midazolam 0.1 mg/kg is appropriate in the elderly patient, 0.05 mg/kg if the patient is compromised by severe comorbid disease.

III. The difficult or failed airway

Blind nasotracheal intubation in the elderly has a higher morbidity rate, particularly from bleeding and posterior pharyngeal perforation; therefore this technique should be used with caution, if at all, in the elderly. When elderly patients have a failed airway, alternatives are similar to those for younger patients. Devices such as the Combitube or laryngeal mask airway are reasonable alternatives in failed-airway situations, as are lighted stylets and fiberoptic devices. Finally, if necessary, surgical cricothyrotomy is always an alternative in the failed-airway situation in any adult, regardless of age.

ADDITIONAL READING

Beers MH, Storrie M, Lee G. Potential adverse drug interactions in the emergency room. *Ann Intern Med* 1990;112:61.

DeMaria EJ. Evaluation and treatment of the elderly trauma victim. *Clin Geriatr Med* 1993;9:461.

Knuddon MM, Lieberman J, Morris JA Jr, et al. Mortality factors in geriatric blunt trauma patients. *Arch Surg* 1994; 129:448.

Lamy PP. Pharmacotherapeutics in the elderly. *Mod Med J* 1989;39:144.

26

Foreign Body in the Adult Airway

Ron M. Walls

Chairman, Department of Emergency Medicine, Brigham and Women's Hospital;
Associate Professor of Medicine, Division of Emergency Medicine,
Harvard Medical School, Boston, Massachusetts

Management of the suspected or known foreign body in the adult airway follows similar rationale to that used in the pediatric patient. The path chosen will depend on the patient's presentation, especially whether the foreign body is causing complete or only partial obstruction and the setting of care.

I. Clinical presentation

The patient with a foreign body in the upper airway will present with signs of upper-airway obstruction. The obstruction may be complete, as in the patient who aspirates a food bolus and cannot move any air or phonate. Although these patients will usually receive treatment in the prehospital setting, they may occasionally present at the emergency department (ED). In addition, a partially obstructing foreign body may be transformed to a completely obstructing foreign body just before ED arrival. A partially obstructing foreign body will cause symptoms of partial upper-airway obstruction, specifically stridor or other audible signs of airway obstruction, subjective difficulty breathing, and often a sense of fear, panic, or impending doom on the part of the patient. In many cases, there will be a preceding condition that has increased the risk of aspiration. Many patients who aspirate food are intoxicated, mentally handicapped, or demented. There may be a history of abnormal swallowing or feeding problems. In some cases, a clear history of the foreign-body incident may be obtained from a bystander or through prehospital providers.

II. Management

Management of the foreign body in the adult airway depends on the location of the foreign body and whether the obstruction is incomplete or complete. The obstruction may be supraglottic, infraglottic, or distal to the carina, and it may be complete or incomplete. Because the precise location of the foreign body is often unknown, the following discussion will focus on the approach to the foreign body whose location is uncertain. In cases where the foreign body has moved distal to the carina, the presentation will not be one of upper-airway obstruction, but rather of increasing respiratory compromise based on the obstruction of one lung or the other. Small foreign bodies, such as aspirated teeth, may move quite far distally in the bronchial tree but may not cause dramatic symptoms.

A. Incomplete obstruction by a foreign body

When a patient presents with an incompletely obstructing foreign body, the most important consideration is to prevent the conversion of a partial obstruction into a complete obstruction. If the patient is breathing spontaneously and oxygen saturation is adequate (or can be made adequate through the use of supplemental oxygen), then the best approach may be to evaluate carefully for the location of the foreign body and to plan for removal in the operating room. For example, if there is an incompletely obstructing foreign body just proximal to the glottis, attempts at removal in the ED might result in displacement of the foreign body into the trachea. The foreign body is then no longer amenable to removal with common ED instruments. Although a fiberoptic bronchoscope may be present in the ED, this is not always satisfactory for foreign-body removal and requires considerable time and expertise in any case. Once a foreign body has traversed the vocal cords and entered the trachea, rigid bronchoscopy is often required. In settings in which transfer to the operating room is not a reasonable option, the best approach is to handle the airway much as one would handle a difficult intubation. Appropriate equipment should be assembled, the patient should be fully preoxygenated, and, following explanation of the procedures, the patient should be given titrated sedation to render him or her amenable to direct laryngoscopy. Topical anesthesia spray may be very helpful as well. With the patient sedated and placed in a slightly head-down position, the operator carefully begins to insert the laryngoscope with the left hand while holding a pair of Magill forceps in the right hand. In this case, the laryngoscope is moved very gently back over the tongue in stepwise fashion to ensure that the foreign body is not pushed further down by the tip of the laryngoscope. The laryngoscope should only be advanced into areas that can be entered with direct visualization. The technique is one of "lift and look" followed by a small advance (perhaps 1 cm), then another "lift and look," and so on. It may be necessary to take a break to allow the patient to reoxygenate. If a foreign body is seen, it is important to look carefully at it prior to attempting removal with Magill forceps. Only after one has determined that the foreign body is amenable to removal with the Magill forceps should this be attempted. Some foreign bodies, especially balls, cannot be grasped well with the Magill forceps. It is often valuable to have a gynecologic tenaculum or a towel clip readily available for such cases. If the foreign body can be grasped and successfully removed, then laryngoscopy should again be performed to ensure that no foreign body remains in the airway. The patient should then be observed for 12 to 24 hours to ensure that there are no pulmonary complications and that no foreign body moved distally in the airway. Chest radiograph may be helpful.

If the foreign body, as identified, does not appear to be amenable to removal with Magill forceps or a tenaculum, then consideration should be given to other means of removal. One possibility is to pass a Foley catheter with a 30-cc balloon distal to the foreign body, inflate the balloon, and use it to dislodge the foreign body upward. Great caution must be taken in doing this, as all such maneuvers may dislodge the foreign body distally, particularly when one is attempting to pass the Foley catheter prior to the attempt at removal. A vascular clamp or hemostat, a towel clip, or any of several other instruments might also be helpful in removing the difficult foreign body. If it is determined that the foreign body will not be amenable to removal from above, despite the consideration of several alternative implements, then it should be removed in an operating room. If this requires transfer of the patient to another facility, the transfer should be done as a critical care transport with either qualified critical care transport personnel or a physician in attendance. In addition, discussion should be held with the receiving hospital regarding whether a preemptive cricothyrotomy ought to be performed. If the foreign body has been visualized above the vocal cords but is in danger of displacement during transport, then a cricothyrotomy to maintain and protect the airway may be advisable. Such decisions have to be individualized and should be made in consultation with the receiving hospital. In cases where the patient can be transferred to the operating room within the same hospital, the only issue is timing. An upper-airway foreign body without complete obstruction should be considered a genuine emergency and all attempts must be made to expedite the patient's transfer to the operating room for definitive management of the foreign body. If the patient's airway becomes completely obstructed while waiting for definitive therapy, then the patient will be managed in a manner identical with that described in the following section.

B. Complete obstruction of the airway

Call for help early. The foreign body may require fiberoptic bronchoscopy or rigid bronchoscopy for removal and the appropriate personnel should be alerted as soon as the situation is identified. When airway obstruction is complete, the patient will be unable to breathe or phonate. This inability to phonate is an important sign of complete upper-airway obstruction, and any phonation at all by the patient indicates incomplete obstruction of the upper airway. The patient with complete airway obstruction will often hold his anterior neck with one or both hands in the "universal choking sign." The patient may appear terrified and will be making attempts at inspiration. In addition, the patient may point to his or her mouth. In general, after complete obstruction of the airway with ensuing apnea, oxygen saturation will fall to levels incompatible with consciousness within a minute or so. Management differs according to whether the patient is conscious or unconscious. If the patient is conscious, the correct initial treatment is proper application of the Heimlich maneuver, which should be repeated until the foreign body is expelled or the patient loses consciousness. There is no point in attempting instrumented removal of a completely obstructing upper-airway foreign body while the patient is still conscious. If the Heimlich maneuver is successful in removing the foreign body and the patient can phonate and breathe normally, then observation for 12 to 24 hours is advised. It is not mandatory to visualize the airway with a laryngoscope or fiberoptic scope unless there is concern about a remaining foreign body. If the Heimlich maneuver is unsuccessful in removing the foreign body and the patient loses consciousness or if the patient presents unconscious with an upper-airway foreign body, then the first step is direct laryngoscopy. Generally, the patient will be flaccid and it will be unnecessary to administer a neuromuscular blocking agent. However, this presentation is analogous to the "crash airway," and it may be necessary to administer a single dose of succinylcholine to achieve sufficient relaxation to identify and remove the foreign body. In any case, under direct laryngoscopy, a foreign body above the glottis should be easily identifiable. With complete obstruction, immediate removal is mandatory, and it is inappropriate to consider transfer to the operating room or any other venue for further care. Again, Magill forceps, tenaculum, towel clip, or any other device can be used to attempt to remove the foreign body. If the foreign body cannot be removed, immediate cricothyrotomy is indicated. After removal of the foreign body, direct laryngoscopy is again performed to ensure that there is no residual foreign body in the upper airway. As the foreign body is removed, the patient may begin spontaneous ventilation immediately or may require a period of bag-and-mask ventilation. This underscores the importance of the "second look" after removal of the foreign body to ensure that there is no additional foreign body in the upper airway before beginning positive-pressure ventilation with a bag and mask. If bag-and-mask ventilation is initiated while a foreign body is still above the glottis, the pressure may force the foreign body below the glottis, where it is too distal to be removed with conventional laryngoscopy.

The laryngoscopy to remove the foreign body should be performed quickly and efficiently. If no foreign body is identified and if the glottis is clearly visualized, then the foreign body must be below the vocal cords. In this case, the first step would be to attempt bag-and-mask ventilation. Ventilation pressures will be high, and this will undoubtedly require a two-person, two-handed technique to try to achieve adequate mask seal and ventilation. If ventilation is successful, it should be continued and the patient should be transferred to the operating room for rigid bronchoscopy. Alternatively, an experienced fiberoptic endoscopist could attempt fiberoptic bronchoscopy in the ED. If bag-and-mask ventilation is unsuccessful in ventilating the patient, then the foreign body must be considered to be completely obstructing the trachea below the vocal cords. In such cases, bag ventilation will be impossible because of high ventilation pressures and it will be obvious to the operator that ventilation pressures are extremely high and that no air is moving. In such cases, the next step is immediate endotracheal intubation and the endotracheal tube should be passed all the way to the 30-cm mark at the teeth so that the obstructing foreign body in the trachea might be pushed down into the right mainstem bronchus. The tube is then withdrawn to its normal level and suctioned, and ventilation is attempted. The strategy here is to try to convert an obstructing tracheal foreign body (which will be lethal) to an obstructing right mainstem bronchial foreign body (which can be removed in the operating room). Thus the patient can be kept alive by ventilating one good lung while the other is obstructed. In such cases, the operator must continually observe the patient for possible development of pneumothorax because ventilation pressures in the proximal airway and the functioning lung will be very high. If the intubation is successful in pushing the foreign body into the right mainstem bronchus and establishing ventilation, then the patient should be transferred to the operating room for definitive care as a true airway emergency. If the maneuver is unsuccessful in establishing a right mainstem bronchus foreign body and the foreign body remains in the trachea, the patient will be irretrievable unless an endoscopist can remove the foreign body within a few minutes. This is an important concept because it underscores the value of alerting endoscopists and otolaryngologists or general surgeons as early as possible when airway foreign body is identified in presentation.

III. Outcome

If the foreign body is successfully removed before hypoxic brain damage occurs, the patient's outcome can be very rewarding. Although there are occasional short-term complications related to the aspiration of the foreign body, such as pneumothorax, aspiration pneumonia, airway edema, or airway trauma, these are generally self-limited and the patient may be anticipated to make a full recovery. If obstruction is not relieved in time, hypoxic brain injury or death will ensue.

IV. Tips and pearls

- If the obstruction is incomplete, move slowly and deliberately to ensure that you do not convert an incomplete obstruction into a complete obstruction.
- Call for help early.
- If the obstructing foreign body is above the vocal cords and cannot be removed, immediate cricothyroidotomy is indicated.
- If the obstructing foreign body is distal to the vocal cords and cannot be seen from above by direct laryngoscopy, cricothyrotomy will be of no benefit and should not be performed.
- The Heimlich maneuver is a reasonable first step in any case of complete obstruction.

ADDITIONAL READING

Chen CH, Lai CL, Tsai TT, et al. Foreign body aspiration into the lower airway in Chinese adults. *Chest* 1997; 112:129–133.

Jones TM, Luke LC. Life threatening airway obstruction: a hazard of concealed eating disorders. *J Accid Emerg Med* 1998;15:332–333.

Kelly SM, Marsh BR. Airway foreign bodies. *Chest Surg Clin N Am* 1996;6:253–276.

Odelowo EO, Komolafe OF. Diagnosis, management and complications of oesophageal and airway foreign bodies. *Int Surg* 1990;75:148–154.

Walls RM. Airway management. In: Rosen P, Barkin R, Danzl DF, et al., eds. *Emergency medicine: concepts and clinical practice,* 4th ed. St Louis: Mosby, 1998.

Yamamoto S, Suzuki K, Itaya T, et al. Foreign bodies in the airway: eighteen-year retrospective study. *Acta Otolaryngol* (Stockh) 1996;525:6–8 (suppl).

27

Airway Management in the Prehospital Setting

Ron M. Walls

*Chairman, Department of Emergency Medicine, Brigham and Women's Hospital;
Associate Professor of Medicine, Division of Emergency Medicine,
Harvard Medical School, Boston, Massachusetts*

Many of the principles of prehospital airway management are identical to those of management in the emergency department (ED). However, local protocols, the availability or unavailability of neuromuscular blocking agents, limited equipment, limited backup, and mandatory transportation of the patient all introduce considerations and issues that are different from those in the ED.

I. The decision to intubate

The decision to intubate the patient in the prehospital setting is based on the same principles as those applied in the ED (Chapter 1). A prehospital algorithm for the decision to intubate is shown in Fig. 27.1. The initial step is a quick evaluation of the patient, with a particular focus on assessment of the airway and ventilation. If the patient is maintaining the airway, protecting the airway, and ventilating and oxygenating adequately, then intubation will rarely be indicated in the prehospital setting. However, failure to maintain or protect the airway or to exchange gases adequately mandates intubation unless the problem can be corrected by other means.

A. Is the patient maintaining the airway?

If the patient is not maintaining his or her own airway, as evidenced by obstructed or noisy breathing, deep coma with unresponsiveness, or apnea, then the airway should be immediately repositioned using the jaw-thrust maneuver to attempt to establish a patent upper airway. Unless the patient has a contraindication to manipulation of the head and neck (e.g., blunt trauma with possible cervical spine injury), the head should be extended on the neck and the mandible should be thrust forward by pressure applied bilaterally at the angles of the mandible. This is best done using the ring or small fingers of the rescuer's hands, so that the remaining fingers can be free to apply and properly seal a mask for ventilation. If the patient does not begin breathing spontaneously when the jaw-thrust maneuver is applied, then bag-and-mask ventilation should be initiated. Placement of nasal and oral airways in the patient will greatly facilitate bag-and-mask ventilation. In most circumstances, bag-and-mask ventilation in this setting should be followed by endotracheal intubation as soon as adequate preparations have been made. If bag-and-mask ventilation is unsuccessful, despite careful attention to proper technique, then immediate intubation is indicated.

195

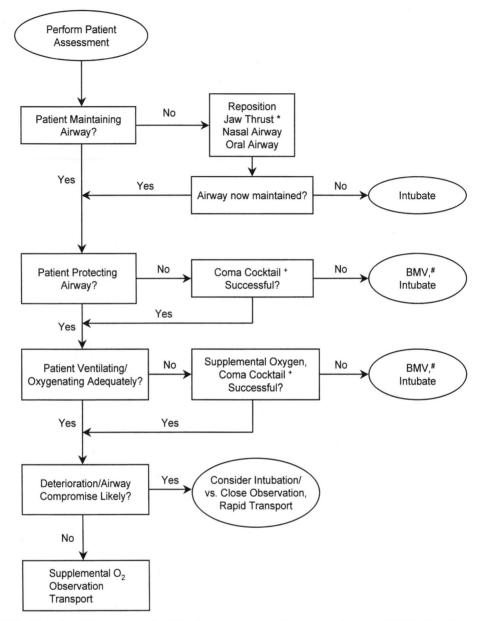

FIG. 27.1. Decision to intubate. *Caution in trauma. [+]Naloxone, glucose. [#]BMV = Bag/Mask Ventilation.

B. Is the patient protecting the airway?

After a patent airway has been established, the next evaluation should determine whether the patient is protecting the airway from aspiration. Aspiration of gastric contents is a serious adverse event and must be prevented. Failure to maintain a patent airway usually indicates loss of protective airway reflexes. It is appropriate to administer a "coma cocktail," which typically includes naloxone in doses of 0.4 to 2.0 mg as a specific reversal agent for opioid overdose, and glucose 25 g for possible hypoglycemia.

In some systems, point-of-care glucose testing is performed rather than empiric glucose administration. If the coma cocktail is unsuccessful in reversing the patient's coma and permitting self-protection of the airway, then bag-and-mask ventilation and intubation are indicated.

C. Are ventilation and oxygenation adequate?

If the patient is maintaining and protecting the airway, the next assessment is of the adequacy of ventilation and oxygenation. If the patient is hypoventilating and a coma cocktail has not already been administered, this should now be done. Oxygenation failure, such as in pulmonary edema, may respond simply to supplemental oxygen via a nonrebreather mask. If neither supplemental oxygen nor administration of reversal agents can establish adequate oxygenation, then bag-and-mask ventilation is indicated, followed by intubation.

D. Other considerations

Finally, there is a population of patients for whom intubation may be indicated despite adequate airway maintenance and protection, and acceptable levels of oxygenation and ventilation. An example would be a pulmonary edema patient who is rapidly tiring but is maintaining oxygen saturations at 90%. If long transport time to the hospital is anticipated and the patient is not responding to other interventions, then intubation may be appropriate prior to development of frank hypoxemia. Other examples might include a patient with drug overdose and rapidly decreasing level of consciousness, the cyclic antidepressant overdose patient who has had a generalized seizure, or certain cases of upper-airway trauma in which ongoing airway bleeding or expansion of a hematoma might threaten the patient. In such cases, careful evaluation and consultation with medical control is essential. In most circumstances, rapid transport of the patient with supplemental oxygen via a nonrebreather mask would be the appropriate course of action. Nevertheless, in certain circumstances, intubation may be both prudent and indicated (Fig. 27.1).

II. Intubation in the prehospital setting

Once a decision to intubate is made, the next step is to choose the best method for intubation, based on individual patient circumstances and the attributes of the Emergency Medical Services (EMS) system and the intubator. The choice will depend on whether neuromuscular blockade is available in the system and whether prehospital cricothyrotomy is possible and permitted, along with a number of individual operator attributes.

If the patient is unresponsive and exhibits agonal cardiac or respiratory activity, the situation is analogous to the crash airway scenario depicted in Chapter 3. The choice to be made here is between oral tracheal intubation and blind nasotracheal intubation. In either case, the patient should have an airway established and oxygenation maintained using a bag and mask until intubation is attempted. If the patient has a relatively clear upper airway (no trauma, no foreign body, and no obstruction) and is breathing spontaneously, then blind nasotracheal intubation may be reasonable. However, apnea is a strong contraindication to blind nasotracheal intubation because the patient's breath sounds are used to guide the tube into place. Similarly, either abnormal anatomy or a foreign body in the upper airway is a strong relative contraindication to this technique. In addition, blind nasotracheal intubation has a lower success rate and higher complication rate than oral intubation. Nevertheless, in some systems and in certain patients, blind nasotracheal intubation may clearly be the preferable method. This may be especially true if the patient's jaw is clenched and the use of neuromuscular blockade is not an option. Also, blind nasotracheal intubation may be a better choice if the patient is relatively inaccessible (e.g., trapped in an automobile) (see later).

Oral intubation via direct laryngoscopy is also an acceptable method for the unresponsive patient and is the method of choice if the patient's jaw is not clenched. In the case of the unresponsive patient, intubation proceeds exactly as described earlier in discussions of the crash airway scenario. Direct laryngoscopy is performed and the tracheal tube is placed under direct vision. If direct laryngoscopy is unsuccessful in visualizing the vocal cords, then a drug-assisted intubation is required. In some settings drug-assisted intubation will include both induction (sedative) agent and neuromuscular blockade. In other settings, where neuromuscular blockade is not permitted, drug-assisted intubation will be done with sedation alone. In either case, drug-assisted intubation may be preferable to blind nasotracheal intubation even in the clenched-jaw patient.

If the patient is conscious and combative and requires intubation, then drug-assisted intubation is indicated. Combative or uncooperative behavior is a strong relative contraindication to blind nasotracheal intubation because of the increased risk of complications in attempting to insert the tube in a patient who is resisting. If the patient is not frankly comatose and is not uncooperative or combative, then assessment must be made as to whether the patient would tolerate laryngoscopy. If the patient is sufficiently cooperative or obtunded to permit oral laryngoscopy without medications, then this may be attempted. Again, preference is expressed for oral intubation over nasal intubation except in circumstances in which the jaw is clenched, thus preventing oral access. Even in such cases, oral intubation with medication may be preferable to blind nasotracheal intubation.

III. Methods of intubation
A. Blind nasotracheal intubation

Blind nasotracheal intubation is discussed in detail in Chapter 8. In general, although blind nasotracheal intubation has been very widely used in prehospital care, it is gradually falling out of favor as medications are being introduced to facilitate intubation in the prehospital setting. Blind nasotracheal intubation has two main uses. First, in circumstances in which direct laryngoscopy and visualization of the glottis would be impossible, blind nasotracheal intubation may be the method of choice. An example would be the patient who is trapped in the automobile after a motor vehicle crash and requires intubation before extrication can be accomplished. In such cases, blind nasotracheal intubation may be the only method that can be used by an operator either from inside or outside the vehicle. The second circumstance is the patient with a clenched jaw. A small number of patients will have increased masseter tone and hence a clenched mandible, even when they are deeply unconscious and breathing inadequately. In such cases, the choice is between administering medications for oral intubation or performing blind nasotracheal intubation. In certain circumstances, blind nasotracheal intubation may be preferable or may be the procedure of choice for the individual operator. Even in such cases, however, administration of medications for a controlled drug-assisted intubation may be preferable to a blind attempt at nasotracheal intubation.

In general, blind nasotracheal intubation should not be performed in patients with asthma, chronic obstructive pulmonary disease, or pulmonary edema unless drug-assisted intubation is impossible. In such patients, prolonged attempts at nasotracheal intubation impair oxygenation and can worsen existing hypoxemia and lead to full-scale respiratory arrest. Again, this is a judgment call and an individual provider might choose to attempt nasotracheal intubation on the patient with status asthmaticus; however, great caution must be exercised, as prolonged or traumatic attempts may worsen the patient's condition.

B. Drug-assisted intubation

Oral intubation is performed using direct laryngoscopy. In some patients, direct laryngoscopy will not be possible unless medications are administered. These medications can take two main forms:

1. Sedation alone
2. Sedation with neuromuscular blockade

A small but increasing number of prehospital systems are using neuromuscular blockade to facilitate intubation in the field. Helicopter flight systems and critical care transport teams are usually trained and experienced in the use of neuromuscular blockade for intubation. Field protocols for sedation or sedation with neuromuscular blockade will vary from system to system. In general, sedation is used when the patient is not sufficiently cooperative with intubation, when mandibular relaxation is felt to be inadequate, or when the jaw is clenched. In such cases, sedative agents such as midazolam, diazepam, lorazepam, or others are administered and titrated until the patient can be intubated. In systems using neuromuscular blockade, typically a protocol dictates both the indications for and the manner of administration of neuromuscular blockade. In such cases, it is almost always mandatory to administer a sedative agent along with the neuromuscular blocking agent to ensure that the patient is optimized for intubation and that there is no undue physiologic or psychologic stress from the intubation attempts. Prehospital sequences are typically much simpler than those used in the emergency department and pretreatment agents are only infrequently used (Chapter 2). A typical prehospital, drug-assisted intubation protocol using neuromuscular blockade is shown in Box 27.1.

The sequence is simplified in the prehospital setting because the number of options are fewer. Prehospital providers rarely carry a wide array of induction agents and the circumstances are less controlled. Thus the complexity of training prehospital providers regarding use of multiple pretreatment agents and the actual administration of these agents in the prehospital setting may present more problems than provide potential benefit for the patient.

C. New airway devices

Several new devices have been developed that may be useful for airway management in the prehospital setting.

  1. *Laryngeal mask airway (LMA).* The LMA is described in detail in Chapter 9. The LMA is inserted blindly through the oropharynx, and the skill is fairly easy to acquire.

Box 27.1. Simplified rapid sequence intubation for prehospital care

1. Prepare equipment and ensure that the patient is in an appropriate area for intubation.
2. Preoxygenate the patient with nonrebreather mask for at least 3 minutes if possible.
3. Pretreatment drugs—infrequently used. Suggestion: lidocaine 1.5 mg/kg intravenously for head injury, reactive airway disease.
4. Paralysis with sedation—administer sedative drug in adequate dose (example: midazolam 0.3 mg/kg) and neuromuscular blocking agent (example: succinylcholine 1.5 mg/kg).
5. Protection—wait 20 seconds. Apply Sellick's maneuver.
6. Placement—45 seconds after drugs are given, intubate. Confirm endotracheal tube placement, secure tube, transport patient.

Although the LMA does not protect the airway against aspiration, it does provide effective ventilation in virtually every patient into which it is placed. In certain circumstances, the patient can be intubated through the LMA, but this is better left for the ED and probably should not be attempted in the field. The standard LMA is available in both reusable and disposable models for prehospital systems. The disposable model is preferable because the LMA will likely stay with the patient once the patient arrives in the receiving hospital.

2. *The Combitube.* The Combitube was developed for use in difficult or impossible ventilation situations and is described in detail in Chapter 9. Basically, the device is inserted blindly through the oropharynx and placed in the esophagus. Once placed, sequential inflation of an oropharyngeal balloon and an esophageal balloon permits sidestream ventilation through open channels in the side of the tube. The Combitube is also relatively easily learned, is reasonably reliable, and can be inserted into a patient in difficult circumstances, such as from the outside of a vehicle.

3. *Lighted stylet.* The lighted stylet is a method of light-assisted intubation and is discussed in detail in Chapter 9. There has been limited experience with the lighted stylet in the prehospital setting, but the technique is relatively easy to learn and may be a helpful adjunct to direct laryngoscopy for oral tracheal intubation in the field.

D. Failed intubation

Failed intubation in the field should be anticipated by evaluation of the patient for difficult airway attributes as discussed in Chapter 5. If a difficult airway is anticipated, it may be most prudent to transport the patient rapidly to the ED for definitive care rather then to spend a prolonged period of time attempting to intubate in the field, perhaps ending in a failed intubation. Transport time should also be taken into consideration when determining whether it is appropriate to perform drug-assisted intubation. Again, in many settings, especially urban systems with short transport times, transport to the ED may be preferable to struggling with a difficult airway in the prehospital setting.

The primary rescue device for failed intubation is bag-and-mask ventilation. Prehospital providers must be expert at bag-and-mask ventilation using both one-handed and two-handed techniques. If bag-and-mask ventilation is inadequate at providing effective oxygenation, the patient should be repositioned, the jaw thrust should be applied vigorously, oral and nasal airways should be placed, a two-handed technique should be used to seal the mask to the patient, and any other steps should be taken that the operator determines might be helpful (Chapter 6). Again, meticulous bag-and-mask ventilation and rapid transport might be the appropriate action if oxygenation is adequate and intubation appears difficult or impossible.

If intubation is unsuccessful, it is important to try to determine why. Chapter 6 describes the sequence of steps involved in successful direct laryngoscopy. Repositioning of the patient, a change in equipment, or even a change in operator may help. In addition, prehospital providers should be familiar with techniques such as the BURP (backward, upward, rightward, pressure on the larynx) maneuver that may facilitate direct laryngoscopy and intubation.

Some systems will allow cricothyrotomy to be performed in the prehospital setting. If this is the case, adequate training and skill maintenance are important. Cricothyrotomy in the field should be an exceedingly rare event. Cricothyrotomy accounts for only approximately 1% of all ED intubations, and although use has varied in reports among various systems, one might anticipate a similar percentage in the field.

E. Tips and pearls

Always weigh the risks and benefits of intubation in the prehospital setting against transport to the ED. In many circumstances, rapid transport might be the best way of managing the airway.

Master bag-and-mask ventilation. There are very few airway emergencies in the prehospital setting that will not be temporized or managed adequately with proper bag-and-mask ventilation until the patient can be transported to hospital.

If transport times are long, especially in systems with high rates of trauma, consider introducing neuromuscular blockade into the prehospital setting. This requires a comprehensive program, including quality oversight.

Newer devices such as the LMA and Combitube may have a role in prehospital care. These should be evaluated on a system-by-system basis.

ADDITIONAL READING

Balk R. The technique of orotracheal intubation. *J Crit Illness.* 1997;12:316–323.

Benumof JL. Difficult laryngoscopy: obtaining the best view. *Can J Anesth* 1994;41:361–365.

Benumof JL. Nonintubation management of the airway: mask ventilation. In: Benumof J, ed. *Airway management: practice and principles.* St Louis: Mosby, 1996:228–254.

Takahata O, Kubota M, Mamiya K, et al. The efficacy of the "BURP" maneuver during a difficult laryngoscopy. *Anesth Analg* 1997;84:419–421.

Walls RM. Airway management. In: Rosen P, Barkin R, Danzl DF, et al., eds. *Emergency medicine: concepts and clinical practice,* 4th ed. St Louis: Mosby, 1998.

Monitoring and Mechanical Ventilation

28

Noninvasive Ventilatory Support in the Emergency Department

Charles V. Pollack, Jr.

*Department of Emergency Medicine, Maricopa Medical Center
and Arizona Heart Hospital, Phoenix, Arizona*

The use of intensive ventilatory support—both noninvasive and invasive—has only recently become an accepted part of emergency department (ED) patient management. Many emergency physicians are increasingly comfortable with initiating mechanical ventilation after intubating the patient in acute respiratory distress. Managing such patients *noninvasively,* however, is often a more unfamiliar approach. Taken to the lowest common denominator, noninvasive ventilatory support (NIVS) with continuous positive airway pressure (CPAP), bilevel positive airway pressure (BL-PAP or Bi-PAP™ [Respironics, Inc]), or mask mechanical ventilation (MMV) merely involves substituting a mask for an endotracheal tube as the physical interface between the ventilator and the patient. The important issues in successfully using NIVS in the ED are those of patient selection and appropriate aggressiveness of therapy—that is, before resorting to endotracheal intubation and mechanical ventilation.

This discussion appears in a manual of airway management because NIVS is sometimes an alternative to ventilatory management in patients with patent airways. A patient without a secure airway is *not* a candidate for NIVS.

I. Indications for noninvasive ventilatory support.

The indications for NIVS in the ED are straightforward: The eligible patient has a patent, nonthreatened airway; is conscious and cooperative; and has an existing—though insufficient—ventilatory drive. If the patient has a threat to his airway, NIVS is contraindicated. If the patient is apneic, NIVS is contraindicated. (BL-PAP and MMV can actually deliver controlled mechanical ventilation via mask; it is unwise to attempt this level of support in the ED, where one-on-one nursing care is ordinarily unavailable.) Patients who may benefit from NIVS may be hypercarbic, hypoxemic, or both. Typical ED patients who should be considered eligible include patients with chronic obstructive pulmonary disease or congestive heart failure (CHF) exacerbation, pneumonia, status asthmaticus, or mild postextubation stridor.

The objectives of NIVS are the same as those of invasive mechanical ventilation: to improve pulmonary gas exchange, relieve respiratory distress, alter adverse pressure/volume relationships in the lungs, permit lung healing, and avoid complications. Patients on NIVS must be monitored as closely as those on ventilators, using familiar parameters (vital signs, arterial blood gasses (ABG), oximetry, chest radiograph, bedside spirometry, etc).

II. Modes of noninvasive ventilatory assistance

Four modes of NIVS are pertinent to emergency medicine, although one is of historic interest only. Intermittent positive-pressure breathing (IPPB) was emergency medicine's first foray into NIVS. The IPPB ventilators are used with either a face mask or a mouthpiece, sense inspiratory effort. and provide a quick burst of pressure to a preset level, augmenting tidal volume (V_t). This pressure is not sustained and inspiration assist is terminated when the preset pressure is reached. There is no CPAP, and the duration of each IPPB treatment was generally limited to 15 to 20 minutes.

Beta-adrenergic-agonist aerosols were given to patients with acute bronchospasm under the presumption that IPPB would (1) reduce work of breathing (WOB), (2) deliver aerosolized particles more deeply into the respiratory tree than by passive inhalation alone, and (3) help clear mucoid secretions. In fact, in controlled studies, IPPB accomplished none of these objectives. It is also expensive in terms of initial equipment purchase, supplies, and personnel required, and its use was associated with a high incidence of induced barotrauma. Today, it has no role in the ED.

CPAP, on the other hand, has extensive and well-documented utility as a means of NIVS in the ED. Mask CPAP is efficacious as the sole ventilatory support in the treatment of pulmonary edema. Some authors have suggested that CPAP provides benefits during acute asthma exacerbation by reducing inspiratory WOB, mean airway pressures, and air trapping. When it is used in obstructive diseases, however, extrinsic CPAP (or PEEP [positive end-expiratory pressure]) must be provided at a level no higher than intrinsic or auto-PEEP ($PEEP_i$) to be potentially beneficial. Intrinsic PEEP results acutely from improper assisted ventilation (when adequate time is not allowed between breaths for complete exhalation), and already exists at baseline in patients with chronic obstructive pulmonary disease (COPD) or acute asthma exacerbation. The end-expiratory pressure in the alveoli becomes more positive than the positive pressure in the more proximal airways; this phenomenon further compromises hemodynamics, makes inspiratory efforts increasingly less effective, and may precipitate volu/barotrauma. Extrinsic PEEP is postulated to allow respiratory muscles previously employed to maintain $PEEP_i$ to relax and be recruited to participate in inspiratory effort, thereby decreasing WOB.

MMV can be used with virtually any mechanical ventilator mode. Most patients tolerate MMV better than they do intubation and mechanical ventilation. Again, however, if the patient must have the machine to breathe for him, then in the ED—where patients cannot be monitored as intensively as in an ICU—the patient probably should be intubated.

Bilevel PAP (BL-PAP, also referred to as Bi-PAP™) conceptually combines inspiratory pressure-supported ventilation (PSV) and CPAP. Noninvasive BL-PAP ventilators provide differential preset support during spontaneous inspiration (inspiratory positive airway pressure, or IPAP) and expiration (EPAP, expiratory positive airway pressure). The IPAP must be set higher than EPAP, and the difference between the two settings is equivalent to the amount of pressure support (PS) provided. BL-PAP is pressure-limited and flow-triggered; the machine senses the initiation of inspiration and immediately cycles to the preset IPAP, thereby increasing V_t with less WOB. IPAP levels are sustained for at least 200 msec and for as long as 3 sec (unlike IPPB), or until the patient ceases inspiratory effort or begins to exhale. The machine then cycles to the EPAP setting, below which it never drops, thereby maintaining supra-atmospheric end-expiratory pressure. The EPAP reduces WOB analogously to PEEP/CPAP.

Although the greatest experience with BL-PAP is in ambulatory nocturnal support, it has the widest potential ED applicability of all modes of NIVS. Its efficacy in acute respiratory failure has been documented in a number of series, although controlled clinical data are lacking. A recent metaanalysis of such trials (Keenan et al, 1997) identified only seven out of 212 that met rigorous inclusion criteria for analysis. Nonetheless, it appears that in selected patients with respiratory distress due to COPD, pulmonary edema, pneumonia, and status asthmaticus, BL-PAP by face or nose mask may often obviate the need for endotracheal intubation and mechanical ventilation. The ventilator is quite portable, with simple controls, and its settings are highly titratable.

III. Invasive versus noninvasive assistance

Patients who need airway protection may be differentiated from those who need intensive ventilatory support. None of the modes of NIVS provide airway protection; when airway patency is not assured, the indication for endotracheal intubation is always present. Once intubated, the patient can be supported, if necessary, with a mechanical ventilator.

Patients with both a patent airway and an intact respiratory drive—even if that drive is clearly insufficient—may be candidates for NIVS. Patients most likely to respond to NIVS in the ED (and therefore avoid intubation) are those with more readily reversible etiologies of their distress, such as COPD exacerbation or high-resistance cardiogenic pulmonary edema. The keys to success with NIVS are to (1) be prepared with adequate equipment and trained personnel in the ED, (2) select and then monitor patients carefully (blood pressure should be normal to preferably high to compensate for the decreased venous return to the heart that results from CPAP/EPAP), (3) treat the underlying condition aggressively and rapidly, and (4) always maintain readiness to intubate the patient if NIVS fails.

The ventilatory management of patients in frank or impending respiratory failure with NIVS is a minute-to-minute, ongoing strategic decision. Noninvasive ventilators (BL-PAP, CPAP) should be readily accessible to the ED, and physicians, nurses, and respiratory care personnel must be comfortable with their use and knowledgeable of their limitations. Patient selection—reliable inclusion parameters for which have not yet been validated—must take into account the overall condition of the patient, the patient's tolerance of mask support versus intubation, and the anticipated degree of reversal of the underlying insult with ventilatory and pharmacologic support. After the decision is made to proceed with a trial of NIVS, preparations for therapeutic failure (i.e., assuring the availability of a laryngoscope, ETT, and bag) must be maintained. Nonventilatory therapy (e.g., diuretics and nitrates for pulmonary edema, beta-adrenergic agonist aerosols and corticosteroids for COPD) must be pursued aggressively. Finally, the patient should be carefully monitored for progress of therapy, tolerance of the mode of support, and any signs of clinical deterioration that indicate a need for definitive ventilatory support. In many patients, noninvasive MMV, mask inspiratory pressure support, or BL-PAP will provide sufficient support of the patient's own ventilatory drive so that more invasive management is unnecessary.

A separate cause for eligibility for NIVS as a primary therapy is the presence of advanced directives regarding limits on resuscitative and life-support procedures. Patients who have prospectively excluded intubation from the treating physician's repertoire should be considered potential candidates for NIVS. Unfortunately, the ethical ramifications of such therapy have been neither fully explored nor resolved. NIVS may be used in this setting either to delay inevitable death with some level of comfort, allowing time for visits with family, or to reverse the underlying acute deterioration from baseline *without* invasive intervention. Whenever possible, informed consent should be sought from the family or power of attorney for such patients before NIVS is initiated.

When NIVS is successful (i.e., when intubation and mechanical ventilation are avoided). several potential therapeutic, patient comfort, and fiscal benefits are derived. The advantages of NIVS vis-à-vis mechanical ventilation include preservation of speech, swallowing, and physiologic airway defense mechanisms; reduced risk of airway injury; reduced risk of nosocomial infection; and probably a decreased length of stay in the intensive care unit because much less weaning of support is necessary.

When compared with intubated and ventilated patients, patients treated with NIVS bear an increased risk of pulmonary barotrauma, aerophagia, and pressure stress to the face (Regarding the latter, BL-PAP is a leak-tolerant system, so pressure sores are a much less frequent complication of extended BL-PAP support than of CPAP or MMV.) In some published series, patients successfully supported in the ED with NIVS are frequently able to be admitted to telemetry units instead of intensive care units, thereby incurring a significant cost savings. Uncontrolled studies without definitive inclusion criteria have found NIVS successful in avoiding intubation and mechanical ventilation in 60% to 90% of the variety of patients on whom it has been clinically tested. This broad range reflects in part the inconsistent inclusion criteria applied by the various authors.

IV. Use in the ED

Recommended initial settings for BL-PAP machines in the noninvasive support of patients in respiratory distress or failure are IPAP of 8 cm H_2O and EPAP of 3 cm H_2O, for a pressure support (IPAP minus EPAP) of 5 cm H_2O. Either a face mask or a nose mask can be used, but a nose mask is generally better tolerated. There are different masks, and the respiratory therapist will measure the patient to ensure a good fit. The flow of supplemental oxygen into the circuit should be governed by pulse oximetry, corroborated by ABG results as necessary; It is appropriate to initiate therapy with 2 to 5 L/min, but this should be adjusted with each titration of IPAP or EPAP. The ventilator should be in spontaneous mode to support the patient's respiratory effort.

As the patient's response to ventilatory and other therapy is monitored (using cardiac and blood pressure monitors, ABGs and oximetry, and the patient's own voiced assessment of tolerance and progress), support pressures are titrated. In one study that achieved 86% success in avoiding intubation among patients in impending or frank respiratory failure caused by a variety of insults, hypoxemic patients were titrated by raising EPAP in 2 cm H_2O steps with IPAP remaining at a fixed interval higher. Hypercapnic patients were managed by raising IPAP in 2 cm H_2O steps with EPAP being increased in a ratio to IPAP of approximately 1:2.5. The $PEEP_i$ cannot be measured by a noninvasive ventilator, so EPAP should generally be maintained below 8 to 10 cm H_2O to be certain that it does not exceed $PEEP_i$ in patients with obstructive lung disease. The IPAP must always be set higher than EPAP.

Patients treated in the ED with NIVS generally should not be given sedatives or major analgesics, since preservation of respiratory drive is essential to the use of these modes. Anecdotally, some physicians who have used BL-PAP extensively report safe use of small, incremental doses of benzodiazepines for patients who have difficulty tolerating the face or nose mask.

Use of NIVS in the ED is likely to expand. Although these techniques are utilized commonly in ICUs, they are only now gaining acceptance among emergency physicians. The most promise for benefit to ED patients from NIVS use is simply expanding its application (i.e., wider use of BL-PAP and CPAP to avoid intubation and its attendant complications). Fiscal pressure to avoid unnecessary intubation and ventilation, with attendant long ICU stays, may also drive expansion of this therapy.

Another potential area of development of NIVS is in the treatment of acute asthma. Although inspiratory pressure support for asthma seems reasonable, the application of CPAP or EPAP is less intuitive. Shivaram et al, however, have demonstrated both a decreased WOB and an increased patient comfort level during CPAP support of acute asthma exacerbations. Another study compared the use of a BL-PAP circuit (IPAP = 10 cm H_2O, EPAP = 5 cm H_2O, PS = 5 cm H_2O) with small-volume nebulizers to deliver beta-adrenergic-agonist aerosol therapy to patients with mild to moderate asthma exacerbations. The BL-PAP patients improved more and faster as measured by change in peak expiratory flow rate. Because the mortality from acute asthma when treated conventionally remains unacceptably high, further study in this area is clearly indicated.

V. Tips and pearls

A trial of NIVS in the ED can be challenging, especially for physicians inexperienced in its use. Optimal results are obtained when autonomy is given to respiratory care personnel more comfortable with this approach (e.g., "BL-PAP at 8/3, 4 L oxygen bleed-in, titrate to effect and keep oxygen saturation $\geq 95\%$"). It is preferred that a noninvasive ventilator be physically housed in the ED; if it must be summoned once a patient arrives, the patient probably will have improved significantly or be intubated by the time the machine is available.

ADDITIONAL READING

Keenan SP, Kernerman PD, Cook DJ, et al. Effect of noninvasive positive pressure ventilation on mortality in patients admitted with acute respiratory failure: a meta-analysis. *Crit Care Med* 1997;25:1685.

Meduri GM. Noninvasive positive-pressure ventilation in patients with acute respiratory failure. *Clin Chest Med* 1996; 17:513.

Pollack CV. Mechanical ventilation and noninvasive ventilatory support. In: Rosen P, Barkin R, Danzl DF, et al, eds. *Emergency medicine: concepts and clinical practice,* 4th ed. St Louis: Mosby, 1998.

Pollack CV, Torres M, Alexander L, et al. A feasibility study of Bi-PAP respiratory support in the emergency department. *Ann Emerg Med* 1996;27:189.

Pollack CV, et al. Treatment of acute bronchospasm with beta-adrenergic agonist aerosols delivered by a bilevel positive airway pressure circuit. *Ann Emerg Med* 1995;26:552.

Shivaram U, Miro Am, Cash ME, et al. Cardiopulmonary responses to CPAP in acute asthma. *J Crit Care* 1993;8:87.

Shivaram U, Donath J, Khan FA, et al. Effects of CPAP in acute asthma. *Respiration* 1987;52:157.

29

Mechanical Ventilation

Michael F. Murphy* and Gregory W. Murphy†

*Departments of Emergency Medicine and Anaesthesiology, Queen Elizabeth II
Health Sciences Centre, Dalhousie University, Halifax, Nova Scotia;
†Mallinckrodt, Inc., St. Louis, Missouri

Setting up a ventilator is a task that few emergency physicians do on a daily basis. However, emergency physicians must know how to order and modify ventilation parameters. This chapter will introduce the lexicon of ventilator management. It will also provide simple explanations of how mechanical ventilators interact with patients (the "modes" of mechanical ventilation) and the two primary ways ventilators deliver a breath: volume-control, and pressure-control ventilation.

Spontaneous ventilation draws air into the lungs (negative pressure); mechanical ventilation pushes it in (positive pressure). In either case, the amount of negative or positive pressure required to deliver the breath (tidal volume) must overcome resistance (R) to airflow. Some of the factors contributing to this resistance are features of the gas, such as its viscosity and density. Less viscous and dense gases create less resistance and generally flow more easily. For instance, helium is less dense than nitrogen and produces better flow characteristics through tight orifices, as one might encounter in epiglottitis or laryngeal cancer. Other factors contributing to this resistance to airflow relate to the caliber, length, and degree of branching of the tube the gas is flowing through. In fact, caliber is the most powerful determinant of this resistance to gas flow, resistance being inversely proportional to the fourth power of the radius (R/r^4).

Gas flowing through a branching network of straight tubes, such as the tracheobronchial tree, may be orderly (*laminar*) or disorderly (*turbulent*). Laminar flow produces less resistance than turbulent flow and therefore takes less pressure to move a similar volume of gas per unit of time when flow is laminar. It also takes less effort (work of breathing [WOB]) on the part of the person or the ventilator. Factors that enhance the chances for flow to be laminar include using gases with lower density and viscosity; shorter, wider tubes (e.g., endotracheal tubes [ETTs]); and no branching. There is nothing we can do to alter the branching nature of the tracheobronchial tree! Turbulent flow is also created when the speed or velocity of gas flow is increased. The more turbulence, the higher the pressure needed to get the gas in, and in the case of mechanical ventilators the greater the risk of pneumothorax and other untoward events.

When it comes to mechanical ventilation, the aim is to have the machine deliver each breath as fast as possible, with the least amount of pressure, but not so fast as to create turbulent flow and high pressures. When one is setting a patient up on a ventilator, the initial inspiratory flow rate (peak flow) is generally set at 50 to 60 L/min. As one turns the flow rate up gradually in sequential breaths, the peak pressure also increases gradually. However, at a certain point (the *critical flow*), a small increase in flow rate produces a large jump in peak pressure. Flow has just become turbulent! As the asthmatic on a ventilator gets better (i.e., less bronchospasm airways of larger caliber), the amount of pressure the ventilator must generate to deliver the same tidal volume falls. This is due to two factors that reduce airway resistance (R_{AW}): the increased caliber (radius) of the airways, and the transition from turbulent to laminar flow.

I. Ventilator terminology
The following terms are used in mechanical ventilation:
A. *Tidal volume* (V_t). The tidal volume is the volume of a single breath. It is usually in the range of 10 to 15 ml/kg. Smaller tidal volumes and more rapid rates are often used in restrictive lung diseases because higher tidal volumes in stiff lungs lead to excessive airway pressure. In obstructive lung diseases one sometimes attempts to increase the tidal volume and decrease the rate (i.e. constant minute volume) to allow more time for expiration. The problem is that this often leads to unacceptably high airway pressures impeding venous return to the heart, lowering cardiac output, and risking pneumothorax. The tradeoff is pressure versus volume.
B. *Respiratory rate* (RR) or *frequency* (f). The usual starting respiratory rate is 10 breaths per minute in the adult. It will be much higher in neonates, infants, and small children, and in those conditions where carbon dioxide production is accelerated (e.g., fever, acidosis, and other hypermetabolic conditions). The non–gas-exchanging parts of the respiratory system (dead space) constitute a fixed volume of each tidal breath. The remainder of the volume in each breath participates in gas exchange and constitutes alveolar ventilation. Rapid respiratory rates and small tidal volumes risk ventilating little more than dead space, a particular risk in infants and small children. The tradeoff here is rate versus volume (alveolar ventilation).
C. *Fractional concentration of inspired oxygen* (F_iO_2). This ranges from the concentration of oxygen in room air (0.21 or 21%) to that of pure oxygen (1.0 or 100%). Though it is possible to administer hypoxic mixtures of gases (less than 21%), it is never done intentionally.
D. *Airways resistance* (R_{AW}). Multiple factors contribute to airways resistance and are described earlier. Subtle changes in peak inspiratory flow rates (peak flow) and ETT diameter and length can contribute materially to airways resistance. The intubated, spontaneously breathing patient experiences a substantial increase in WOB as the ETT size is reduced. Try sometime to breathe through a drinking straw. After a short time, air hunger and fatigue become appreciable. The same thing happens to a patient breathing spontaneously through an ETT, especially a small one.
E. *Ventilation mode.* This refers to the way the patient interacts with the ventilator and is of three types (Pattern of breathing):
   • Continuous mechanical ventilation (CMV)
   • Synchronized intermittent mandatory ventilation (SIMV)
   • Continuous positive airway pressure (CPAP)
F. *Volume-control ventilation* (VCV) and *pressure-control ventilation* (PCV) describe how the ventilator controls and delivers a volume of gas, breath by breath.

II. Ventilation modes
Mechanical ventilators usually have three modes of ventilation to chose from: continuous mechanical ventilation (CMV), synchronized intermittent mandatory ventilation (SIMV), and continuous positive airway pressure (CPAP). The mode is picked by the individual selecting and setting the parameters for ventilation, depending on the needs of the patient.
A. *CMV, or assist/control ventilation mode.* This mode is usually selected for patients who have no spontaneous respiratory activity of their own, such as overdoses and those

given long-acting neuromuscular blocking drugs. The patient receives a minimum number of breaths each minute, at a predetermined tidal volume. This is called a *controlled* or *mandatory* breath. If the patient initiates his own inspiration, the negative pressure will trigger the ventilator to deliver a breath at the preset tidal volume, an *assisted* breath. The patient can choose whatever rate he or she prefers, but every breath is that of the preset tidal volume and the rate will not fall below the preset level.

B. *SIMV ventilation mode.* This mode is selected for patients who have some respiratory activity of their own, but you want to ensure that they get a minimum minute ventilation. Patients receive a minimum number of breaths each minute at a predetermined tidal volume (mandatory or assisted breaths). They are also permitted to breathe spontaneously, at a rate greater than that set by the operator, at a volume of their own choosing (spontaneous breaths). This mode is often used when attempting to wean patients from mechanical ventilation. It allows you to get some idea of how adequately they are ventilating on their own while allowing them to build strength in their respiratory muscles to enhance the success of weaning.

C. *CPAP ventilation mode.* This mode is selected for patients who are breathing spontaneously through an endotracheal or tracheostomy tube. It may be selected to predict whether the patient can be safely extubated. It is also used to decrease the WOB through a tube (drinking-straw concept) and in some forms of lung disease. Various forms of pressure support are employed to augment ventilation and oxygenation (by optimizing functional residual capacity). Pressure-supported ventilation (PSV), also called *positive-pressure support* (PPS), can be used to decrease the WOB. When used in this manner the operator selects an amount of pressure (PSV pressure) that the ventilator will supply at the instant the patient begins inspiration. This helps the patient overcome airways resistance and makes it easier to get a breath. The PSV pressure is usually titrated to a value that results in a normal spontaneous tidal volume (5 to 7 ml/kg) or until the patient appears to relax and atrial blood gasses (ABGs) are within an acceptable range. Continuous positive airway pressure (CPAP) may also be called positive end-expiratory pressure (PEEP) when used this way.

III. How the ventilator delivers a breath
  A. Volume-control ventilation
    In this method of delivering a breath the operator sets the tidal volume of each breath. The pressure required to deliver this volume varies, depending on the compliance and resistance of the lungs, the flow rate selected, the size and length of the ETT, and other minor factors as discussed earlier. In adults, the initial peak flow is usually set to 50 to 60 L/min and then adjusted to the *critical flow point,* which is the maximum flow rate at which flow remains mostly laminar. As the flow rate is slowly and steadily increased, a sudden jump in pressure indicates that flow has become turbulent (i.e., the critical flow point). The flow rate is then reduced to just below this point. Pressure alarms are set (usually at 10 to 15 cm/H_2O greater than peak inspiratory pressure [PIP]) to warn of the risk of barotrauma and identify changes in compliance and resistance.

    With VCV, one is also able to determine the flow characteristics of the delivered breaths. The waveform may be square or decelerating (Fig. 29.1). Choosing a square wave will result in the tidal volume being delivered at the constant peak flow selected throughout inspiration. This waveform usually generates a higher peak pressure than the decelerating waveform but has the advantage of a shorter inspiratory time and more time for expiration. A decelerating flow wave will cause inspiration to be initiated at the selected peak flow and then decelerates linearly as the breath is delivered. Because resistance to flow normally increases as the breath is delivered, the decelerating

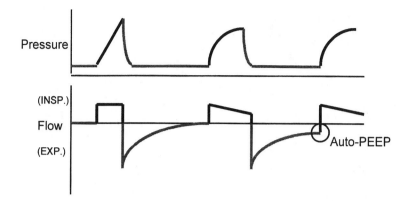

FIG. 29.1. Volume-control ventilation. The lower trace demonstrates a square flow waveform first. The next waveform is a decelerating waveform. Note that the peak pressure generated by the square waveform exceeds that of the decelerating waveform. The third waveform demonstrates inspiration being initiated before expiratory flow has reached zero. This is how breath stacking and auto-PEEP occur.

waveform generally results in lower peak inspiratory pressures. However, this increases the inspiratory time, at the expense of expiratory time, potentially trapping gas in the lung (stacking breaths), and leading to a continuous buildup of pressure called *auto-PEEP*. For this reason, the peak flow setting for decelerating flow wave is ususally higher than that used in a square wave flow pattern. Auto-PEEP may lead to overdistension and rupture of alveoli (volutrauma) and decreased venous return and cardiac output. Most mechanical ventilators will measure auto-PEEP. When setting up the ventilator, one can switch back and forth from one waveform to another in attempting to determine which is best for the patient.

B. Pressure-control ventilation

In this method of delivering a breath, the operator specifies an inspiratory pressure and an inspiratory time (I/E ratio) predicted to give a reasonable rate and tidal volume, based on the patient's expected resistance and compliance. The peak flow of the administered tidal breath and the flow waveform vary according to the patient's resistance and compliance. Early in inspiration the ventilator generates a flow rate that is sufficiently rapid to reach the preset pressure, automatically alters the flow rate to stay at that pressure, and cycles off at the end of the predetermined inspiratory time. The flow waveform created by this method is a decelerating pattern (Fig. 29.2). A normal I/E ratio is 1:2. If the respiratory rate is 10 breaths per minute evenly distributed over the minute, each cycle of inspiration and expiration is 6 seconds. With an I/E ratio of 1:2, inspiration is 2 seconds and expiration is 4 seconds.

The I/E ratio is usually determined by simply observing the pressure and flow waveforms on the ventilator monitor, especially the termination of flow at the end of expiration to avoid generating auto-PEEP (Fig. 29.3). The inspiratory pressure is selected and then the inspiratory time is adjusted by watching the monitor so that when the end inspiratory flow approaches zero, inspiration is terminated and expiration begins. Short inspiratory times lead to low tidal volumes and hypoventilation; long ones may increase mean intrathoracic pressure and compromise hemodynamic function.

In general, pressure-control ventilation imposes less WOB on the patient than volume-control ventilation. Newer ventilators allow the operator to select either op-

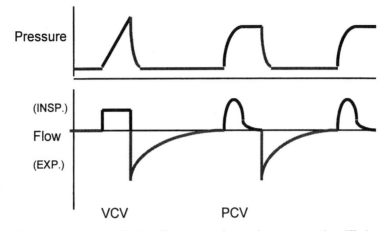

FIG. 29.2. Pressure-control ventilation. These waveforms demonstrate the differing waveform characteristics between VCV and PCV. Note that PCV generates lower peak pressures than VCV.

tion and determine what is best in a given situation. Older ventilators may not. No matter what option is selected, alarms are set to warn of pressures and volumes that are too low or too high.

IV. Initiating mechanical ventilation

Mechanical ventilators simply do for patients what they cannot do for themselves: breathe. The indication for mechanical ventilation is the failure of the patient to maintain adequate gas exchange.

The patient who is spontaneously breathing possesses a complex series of physiologic feedback loops that control the volume of gas moved into and out of the lungs each minute (minute ventilation). They automatically determine the respiratory rate and the volume of each breath necessary to effect gas exchange and maintain homeostasis. The patient who is entirely dependent on a ventilator has no such "servocontrol" mechanism and must rely

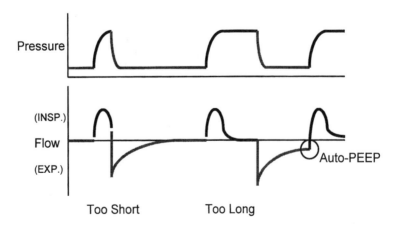

FIG. 29.3. PCV and I/E ratio. The first waveform set demonstrates an inspiratory time that is so short that the tidal volume is likely insufficient. The second and third waveform sets demonstrate how an inspiratory time that is too long may lead to breath stacking and auto-PEEP, as illustrated in Fig. 29.1.

on the individuals setting the ventilatory parameters to meet their needs adequately. In the old days this meant frequent blood gas determinations. Now we rely on noninvasive techniques such as pulse oximetry and end-tidal carbon dioxide monitoring.

A certain amount of ventilation is required each minute (minute ventilation or minute volume) to remove the carbon dioxide produced by metabolism and delivered to the lungs by the circulatory system each minute. This minute volume approximates 100 ml/kg, provided the metabolic rate is normal. Febrile patients, for instance, produce 25% more carbon dioxide each minute than the same patients when they are afebrile. Minute ventilation would need to increase by 25% to accommodate for this, guided by arterial blood gases or end-tidal carbon dioxide monitoring.

In general, we use the rule of 10s in initiating ventilation in an adult:
- V_t – 10 ml/kg
- f – 10 breaths/minute
- F_iO_2 – 1.0

The vast majority of patients are easily ventilated, and this formula produces reasonable arterial blood gas tensions. Larger tidal volumes and lower rates delivering the same minute ventilation are acceptable, provided the volume/pressure tradeoff is acceptable. Similarly, faster rates and smaller tidal volumes are acceptable, provided the rate/volume tradeoff is accounted for.

High airway pressure is a material enemy in mechanical ventilation. The many faces of barotrauma (pneumothorax, pneumomediastinum, etc.) are visible outcomes of high airway pressure. However, this airway pressure is also transmitted directly to the intrathoracic compartment compressing the great veins and the right atrium, and when averaged over the respiratory cycle is known as the *mean intrathoracic pressure*. This compromises cardiac output and may in severe situations, such as that with the ventilated asthmatic, produce a Pulseless Electrical Activity (PEA) rhythm! Airway pressure exceeding 35 to 40 CWP (by convention, airway pressures are measured in CWP, not millimeters of mercury) is generally considered a barotrauma risk, though barotrauma is possible at lower pressures with some disorders. The same applies to mean intrathoracic pressure and venous return.

For some patients, the most perplexing task in establishing adequate mechanical ventilation is trading off rate, volume, and pressure. Ventilating the asthmatic is a good example. On the one hand, the tidal volume has to be sufficient, at a given rate, to provide reasonable minute ventilation. One wants the inspiratory part of the cycle to be short (i.e., rapid peak flow) to allow maximum time for expiration and avoid starting the next inspiration before expiration is complete ("stacking breaths"). Meanwhile, the rate has to be slow enough to allow reasonable time for expiration. The dilemma is how to give a big enough tidal volume, quickly, and not in excess of 40 CWP! Deliberate hypoventilation (permissive hypercapnia) is one strategy employed to attenuate the risks of high airway pressures. In some cases, one simply accepts the risks and acts accordingly. However, this is one case where attention to detail can make a material difference:
- Use as large an ETT as possible;
- cut the ETT to minimize the length;
- adjust the peak flow in an attempt to minimize turbulent flow.

Chapters in Section 4 deal with specific disorders and discuss initiating mechanical ventilation for those conditions.

V. Tips and pearls
- Have a respiratory therapist (RT) review the features of ventilators available for use in your particular ED

- Know how to turn the ventilator on and off, and how to silence the alarms. These minimal steps will preserve calm until the RT can respond. Bag ventilation can be used to deal with temporary problems and provides the additional feedback of "feel"
- Use the rule of 10s to initiate ventilation
- Understand the typical resistance and compliance characteristics of the various respiratory disorders. It may help predict if and how the rule of tens may need to be altered
- Use CMV in totally apneic patients and SIMV for patients with some spontaneous respiratory effort
- Select an intubated patient with relatively normal resistance and compliance, such as an overdose patient. Switch back and forth from volume control to pressure control, if your ventilator has the capability of doing so, to see the difference in peak pressures and waveforms
- Always disconnect the patient from the breathing circuit when moving them. The circuit is heavy and may drag the ETT out, especially in infants and children

30

Monitoring the Emergency Airway Patient

Michael F. Murphy

Departments of Emergency Medicine and Anaesthesiology,
Queen Elizabeth II Health Sciences Centre, Dalhousie University, Halifax, Nova Scotia

Monitors are nothing more than "decision support" aids. The definition of the verb *to monitor* is "to watch, observe or check, especially for a special purpose"; and a definition of the noun *monitor* is "that which warns or instructs." To monitor means to measure or observe a physiologic parameter either continuously or intermittently. The monitoring device may give one a "snapshot in time" or over time allow one to detect deterioration, track improvement, or follow the effects of interventions.

Two monitoring technologies are fundamental to airway management: pulse oximetry and end-tidal carbon dioxide measurement.

I. Pulse oximetry

Pulse oximetry is particularly useful in the ED evaluation of patients with acute cardio-pulmonary disorders such as bronchiolitis, asthma, heart failure, and chronic obstructive pulmonary disease. It is a standard monitoring parameter for patients undergoing sedation and for patients with a decreased level of consciousness, such as intoxication, overdose, and head injury. Its ability to decrease the frequency with which arterial blood gases are done has also been demonstrated. Continuous monitoring may indicate the insidious development of shock as vasoconstriction develops.

Continuous pulse oximetry monitoring is mandatory for patients requiring endotracheal intubation. It has been shown to decrease the incidence and duration of hypoxemic episodes during this procedure. It must be remembered, however, that adequate oxygen saturation does not ensure adequate ventilation, particularly for patients with decreased levels of consciousness.

The pulse oximeter provides a noninvasive and continuous means of rapidly determining arterial oxygen saturation (percent of hemoglobin saturated with oxygen) and its changes. Pulse oximeters are easy to use and interpret, pose no risk to the patient, and are relatively inexpensive. However, a reliable interpretation of the information given by these devices requires an appreciation of their limitations in certain situations.

"Transmission" oximetry is based on differences in the optical transmission spectrum of oxygenated and deoxygenated hemoglobin. At the wavelength of red light (660 nanometers) reduced hemoglobin absorbs about 10 times as much light as oxyhemoglobin, whereas at the infrared wavelength (940 nanometers) absorption is roughly equal. Pulse oximeters measure red and infrared light transmitted through a tissue bed, and in particular the pulse variations in that transmission. In essence, they measure the ratio of oxygenated hemoglobin to the total amount of hemoglobin and present the result as the percent of hemoglobin that is oxygenated.

Oximetry light sources are light-emitting diodes (LEDs) and the detectors are photo-diodes. The light absorption is divided into a pulsatile (AC) component due to the pulsatile arterial blood and a nonpulsatile (DC) component reflecting the tissue bed, including venous and capillary blood and nonpulsatile arterial blood. The pulse oximeter's digital microprocessor first determines the AC component of absorbance at each wavelength and divides this by the corresponding DC component to obtain a "pulse-added" absorbance. It then calculates the ratio of these pulse-added absorbances, a nonlinear but reproducible function of the oxygen saturation of arterial blood. The microprocessor converts this pulse added absorbance to saturation. Data averaged over several arterial pulse cycles are then presented as saturation (SpO_2). There is an excellent correlation between arterial hemoglobin oxygen saturation and pulse oximeter saturation.

In addition to arterial hemoglobin, other absorbers in the light path include skin, soft tissue, and venous and capillary blood. The accuracy of the information is compromised in patients with severe vasoconstriction (e.g., shock, hypothermia), excessive movement, synthetic fingernails and nail polish, severe anemia or the presence of abnormal hemoglobins, such as carboxyhemoglobin (COHb) and methemoglobin (MetHb). Their presence will contribute to light absorption and cause errors in the pulse oximetry readings. The pulse oximeter sees COHb as though it is mostly OxyHb and gives a falsely high reading. MetHb produces a large pulsatile absorbance signal at both the red and infrared wavelengths. This forces the absorbance ratio toward unity, which corresponds to a SpO_2 of 85%. Thus in the presence of high levels of MetHb the SpO_2 is erroneously low when the arterial saturation is above 85% and erroneously high when the arterial saturation is below 85%. In dark-skinned races, erroneously high readings (about 3% to 5%) and a higher incidence of failure to detect signal have been reported.

The pulse oximeter probe is generally placed on a finger or a toe. However, several other types of probes are available to allow placement in other anatomic locations, most commonly the ear lobe and the bridge of the nose. In general, signals are weaker from ears than from fingers, except in the face of hypotension or peripheral vasoconstriction, but ear responses are faster. Nasal bridge probes have been reported to read falsely high in some circumstances.

II. End-tidal carbon dioxide monitoring
A. Quantitative end-tidal carbon dioxide monitoring
1. Capnograph

   Capnography is the graphic record of instantaneous carbon dioxide concentrations (capnogram) in the respired gases during a respiratory cycle (Fig. 30.1). Capnometry is the measurement and display of CO_2 concentrations on a visual display. Both machines usually also display the end-tidal CO_2 concentration numerically.

   The measurement of CO_2 in the expired air is a direct indicator of CO_2 elimination by the lungs. Thus capnography confers an ability to monitor CO_2 production, pulmonary perfusion, and alveolar ventilation, as well as respiratory patterns. The normal capnograph waveform itself (i.e., the trace visible on the monitor) consists of three phases (Fig. 30.1):

   Phase I represents a CO_2-free portion of the respiratory cycle. Most commonly, this is the inspiratory phase, though it may represent apnea or a disconnection of the device from the patient.

   Phase II is the rapid upstroke of the curve representing the transition from inspiration to expiration and the mixing of dead space and alveolar gas.

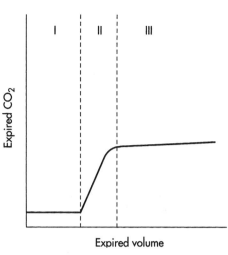

FIG. 30.1 The three phases of the normal capnograph waveform are depicted. (From Murphy MF. Monitoring the emergency patient. In: Rosen P, Barkin R, Danzl DF, et al., eds. *Emergency medicine: concepts and clinical practice,* 4th ed. St Louis: Mosby, 1998, with permission.

Phase III is the "alveolar plateau." This represents alveolar gas rich in carbon dioxide. It tends to slope gently upward, indicating a rising alveolar P_{CO_2}. As inspiration is initiated, detected CO_2 levels rapidly fall back to the Phase I baseline.

B. Types of devices

There are four spectrographic physical methods currently used to measure the concentration of CO_2 in the respiratory gases: infrared, mass, Raman, and photoacoustic spectrography.

1. *Infrared devices* are compact and less expensive than the other devices and are the most common devices in current clinical usage. Carbon dioxide selectively absorbs a specific wavelength of infrared light (4.3 μm). Because the amount of light absorbed is proportional to the concentration of the absorbing molecules, the concentration can be determined by comparing the absorbance with that of a known standard.

2. A *mass spectrograph* separates gases and vapors of differing molecular weights and utilizes differences in weights to determine the concentrations of components in a sample. Mass spectrographers are large and expensive and not appropriate for bedside use at this time.

3. *Raman spectrographs* expose a gas to an argon laser beam. Molecules in the specimen absorb the light, producing unstable vibrational or rotational energy states known as "Raman scattering." The pattern of the scatter is used to determine the types and concentrations of gases in the sample. The Raman technique is gaining popularity and is currently used to identify and quantify gases and vapors used in anesthetic practice.

4. *Photoacoustic spectrography* utilizes an acoustic measuring technique rather than the optical one used in infrared spectrography. The photoacoustic method is based on the same principles as the infrared analyzers, although the methods differ in their measurement technique. Photoacoustic systems are alleged to be more accurate and reliable, and require less frequent maintenance and calibration.

C. Methods of sampling

Capnometers sample the expired gas in one of two ways: sidestream or mainstream.

1. *Sidestream* units aspirate a sample of gas into a measuring chamber in the device itself. These devices have the advantage of being fairly accurate in nonintubated as well as intubated patients. The sampling tubing, however, is small in caliber and may become blocked with water vapor and introduce a source of failure.

2. *Mainstream* units place the measuring device within the breathing circuit. The mainstream devices are useful only in intubated patients, are bulky and heavy, and may burn patients because they must be heated to prevent condensation.

The most popular technology employs a sidestream sample of expired gas drawn by a small sampling catheter into an infrared, sensing chamber.

D. Accuracy

The most popular use of this technology to date in the emergency department is the verification of endotracheal tube placement in the trachea. However, end-tidal CO_2 detection is also useful in other clinical scenarios:

1. Estimating Alveolar partial Pressure of Carbon Dioxide (P_aCO_2) using the end-tidal CO_2. A gradient normally exists between the end-tidal ($P_{et}CO_2$) and arterial PCO_2 (P_aCO_2) values because of the contribution of physiologic dead space. The end-tidal concentration is usually 2 to 5 mmHg less than the arterial reading; however, many emergency department conditions can corrupt this normal gradient. The most common example of this is the ventilated patient with chronic obstructive pulmonary disease or asthma where the slope of Phase III of the capnograph rises steadily because of delayed emptying of alveoli, rather than being relatively flat, as it is normally. In this instance, the next mechanical inspiration may cut the expiratory phase short before the true end-tidal point is reached, thus providing a falsely low end-tidal CO_2. The clinician should be suspicious of any end-tidal reading, where Phase III of the waveform is interrupted or is not relatively flat. This is true in both non-ventilated and ventilated patients. Determining the P_aCO_2 by blood gas analysis and comparing it with the end-tidal reading provides a baseline gradient from which to judge increases and decreases in $P_{et}CO_2$.

2. Detecting accidental extubation. In this circumstance, the capnograph tracing loses its characteristic shape and remains flat at a zero or nearly zero level.

3. Indicating the adequacy of Cardio Pulmonary Resuscitation (CPR) and the return of spontaneous circulation. End-tidal concentration of carbon dioxide depends on several physiologic variables, including pulmonary perfusion. Failure to detect adequate end-tidal CO_2 in a properly intubated cardiac arrest patient is an ominous sign of failure of pulmonary perfusion and gas exchange, and predicts death if it persists. Return of spontaneous circulation (ROSC) will begin to restore pulmonary perfusion and gas exchange, and a more normal capnograph tracing will emerge.

4. Monitoring patients undergoing deep sedation in the emergency department as an indicator of hypoventilation and apnea. Sidestream sampling in spontaneously breathing, nonintubated patients is a reliable technique for end-tidal CO_2 analysis.

5. A correlation between the slope of Phase III of the waveform and forced expiratory volume in 1 second (FEV_1) has been identified in adult asthmatics. This may provide an objective measure of the degree of airway obstruction in patients unwilling or unable to cooperate with the measurement of airflow obstruction (e.g. the intubated and ventilated, and the very young) and may be used to help assess response to therapy.

E. Qualitative end-tidal CO_2 monitoring

Colorimetric devices have been developed that are capable of detecting end-tidal CO_2 and thus indicating intratracheal placement of an endotracheal tube. A pH-sensitive indicator changes color when exposed to carbon dioxide. The color changes from purple (when exposed to room air) to yellow (when exposed to 4% CO_2). The indicator, housed in a plastic device, is inserted between the endotracheal tube and the ventilator bag. The response time of the device is sufficiently fast to detect such changes on a breath-by-breath basis. Electronic qualitative end-tidal CO_2 detectors are also available. These devices sample exhaled gas and indicate, by a light or audio signal, when CO_2 is detected. The advantage to these devices is that some have alarms that will sound if CO_2 detection ceases for more than a few seconds. The devices are expensive but use inexpensive disposable samplers, so ongoing cost is low after initial purchase.

The limitations of qualitative end-tidal CO_2 detectors are particularly evident in the following clinical situations:

1. Metabolic CO_2 production is low (e.g., hypothermia). This may produce an "intermediate" reading. The issue here is the clinician's understanding of CO_2 production, not the reliability of the device.
2. Reduction in pulmonary perfusion as is seen in profound shock and prolonged cardiac arrest. In shock, one may see an intermediate reading. In prolonged cardiac arrest, a false negative (i.e., no CO_2 detection) may occur in some cases even when the tube is in the trachea. Despite this, failure to detect CO_2 in *any* setting should be interpreted as esophageal intubation until tracheal intubation is definitely confirmed. In such circumstances, an aspiration device may provide proof of tracheal or esophageal intubation.

III. Summary

The monitoring technology discussed in this chapter represents significant advances in the airway management and the practice of emergency medicine. The devices are noninvasive, and they provide continuous, real-time measures of physiologic performance. They also have the potential to free staff to attend to other tasks. The real danger is the false sense of security they may impart if the users of the technology are not aware of their limitations.

ADDITIONAL READING

Anderson JA, Vann WF. Respiratory monitoring during pediatric sedation: pulse oximetry and capnography. *Pediatr Dent* 1988;10:94–101.

Aughey K, Hess D, Eitel D, et al. An evaluation of pulse oximetry in prehospital care. *Ann Emerg Med* 1991;20: 887–891.

Bhavani-Shankar K, Moseley H, Kumar AY, et al. Capnometry in anesthesia. *Can J Anaesth* 1992;36:617–632.

Bishop J, Nolan T. Pulse oximetry in acute asthma. *Arch Dis Child* 1991;66:724–725.

Galdun JP, Paris PM, Stewart RD. Pulse oximetry in the emergency department. *Am J Emerg Med* 1989;7:422–425.

Garnett AR, Gervin CA, Gervin AS. Capnographic waveforms in esophageal intubation: effect of carbonated beverages. *Ann Emerg Med* 1989;18:387–390.

Kellerman AL, Cofer CA, Joseph S, et al. Impact of portable oximetry on arterial blood gas test ordering in an urban emergency department. *Ann Emerg Med* 1991;20:130–134.

Murphy MF. Monitoring the emergency patient. In: Rosen P, Barkin R, Danzl DF, et al., eds. *Emergency medicine: concepts and clinical practice,* 4th ed. St Louis: Mosby, 1998:119–123.

Paulus DA. Capnography. *Int Anesthesiol Clin* 1989;27:167–175.

Short L, Hecker RB, Middaugh RE, et al. A comparison of pulse oximeters during helicopter flight. *J Emerg Med* 1989;7:639–643.

Wright SW. Conscious sedation in the emergency department: the value of capnography and pulse oximetry. *Ann Emerg Med* 1992;21:551–555.

Appendix
The Difficult Airway Cart

Robert J. Vissers

*Department of Emergency Medicine, University of North Carolina,
Chapel Hill, North Carolina*

It is recommended that all emergency departments (EDs) have a difficult airway equipment cart. This is one of the most important aspects of the preparation phase in airway management. The equipment within the cart will vary according to the needs and preferences of the particular department and the operators who will be using the cart. There are, however, general principles in its preparation and maintenance that will make the difficult airway cart optimally functional in the stressful circumstances for which it is required.

I. Portable cart

A portable storage unit can hold all the equipment needed to manage the difficult airway. The difficult airway may be precipitant and occasionally unanticipated. Therefore it is essential that the cart be mobile and easy to get to. The cart should be kept in the resuscitation area of the ED or a similarly immediately accessible location. The cart should be durable, with wheels that can be locked, and have a flat working surface approximately 3 feet, 6 inches from the floor. The drawers must be lockable by key. Emergency medical staff must carry a key with them at all times while in the department. Carts are commercially available at a cost of $200 to $400. Sears has an assortment of Mastercraft carts ideally suited for this purpose (Fig. A.1).

II. Cart organization

Clear labeling and cart organization are essential to the function of the cart. All items should be accessible and easily located in a matter of seconds. Each drawer must have a general identifying label on the outside (i.e., "surgical airways"). A more detailed description of drawer contents can be laminated and taped to the top surface. Finally, an informational resource must be created for the cart. Ideally, a binder may be chained to the cart and contain the following information: detailed listing of each drawer, device descriptions and product inserts, instructions for maintenance, restocking instructions, manufacturer listing.

III. Maintenance

There must be a method for automatically restocking the cart as its items are utilized. Many devices are costly and unique to the airway cart and should be labeled to identify them as the property of the ED. Some devices, such as the fiberoptic scopes, require specific cleaning instructions. It is helpful to assign an attending emergency physician to the general design, maintenance, and updating of the cart.

IV. Education

It is essential that all medical staff who may use the cart be intimately familiar with its contents. It is a good idea to have a formal annual review of the cart with the operators to main-

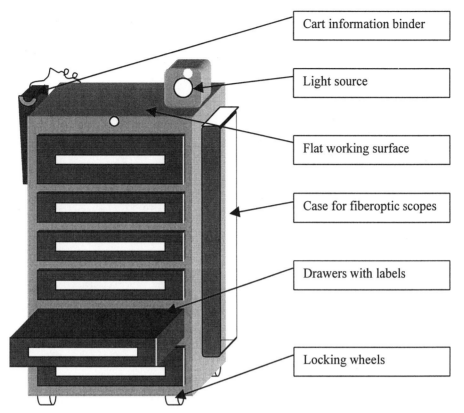

Cart information binder

Light source

Flat working surface

Case for fiberoptic scopes

Drawers with labels

Locking wheels

FIG. A.1. Illustration of a difficult airway cart for the emergency department.

tain familiarization, allow for the introduction of new devices, and provide an opportunity for feedback and improvement. The operators should receive not only initial training in the devices but ongoing education and practice to maintain an adequate skill level.

V. Contents

The contents of the cart will vary with the clinical needs of the department, associated costs, and operator preferences for specific airway devices. In general, there should be a basic intubation kit, a drug kit, nonsurgical rescue airways, surgical airways, devices to improve endotracheal intubation, and preparatory materials. See box A.1 for content lists.

A. Basic intubation kit

Depending on the size of the department, there may be several of these kits in the ED (e.g., in each resuscitation room as well as in the airway cart). We recommend opening the kit on top of the cart and preparing and checking the equipment at the start of each shift. The kits can be kept in a portable bag.

B. Drug kit

Many of the drugs used in a rapid sequence intubation (RSI) can be kept at room temperature and are not restricted, allowing for the creation of a small portable RSI drug kit. A basic RSI kit may contain etomidate, succinylcholine, pancuronium, ketamine, lidocaine, and atropine.

C. Fiberoptic scopes

If you choose to add a fiberoptic scope to your cart, it should be stored in a separate locked metal case attached to the side of the cart. This will help protect these expen-

Box A.1.   A suggested equipment list for a difficult airway cart

Drawer one: Basic airway kit

Cuffed endotracheal tubes, 6.0, 6.5, 7.0, 7.5, 8.0, 8.5 mm	10-ml syringe
Oral airway 80, 90, 100 mm	Colorimetric end-tidal CO_2 detector
Nasopharyngeal airway 28, 30, 32 F	Yankauer suction tip
Bag and mask	Laryngoscope handle
Stylets	Laryngoscope blades, MacIntosh 3 and 4
McGill Forceps	Laryngoscope blades, Miller 2 and 3

Drawer two: Preparation materials

Alcohol prep	Syringes 3×10 ml
Iodine prep	Needles 19, 22, 25 gauge, 1.5 inch
Silicone lubricant	Cetacaine spray
Three-way stopcocks	Neosynephrine 0.5% spray or drops
Gauze 3×3 inch	lidocaine 4% for topical spray
Albuterol multi-dose inhaler	lidocaine 2% viscous jelly
Tongue blades	lidocaine 4% viscous jelly
Sutures, silk, 3-0	lidocaine 1% local anesthetic
Scalpels no. 11	lidocaine 2% local anesthetic
Intravenous catheters, 14-gauge	RSI drug kit

Drawer three: Laryngoscopes and endotracheal tubes, stylets

Laryngoscope blades, MacIntosh 2, 3, 4	Magill forceps, large and small
Laryngoscope blades, Miller 2, 3	Lighted stylet, handle
Laryngoscope handle, short	Lighted stylet, disposable stylets
Laryngoscope handle, regular	Stylets adult
Bullard blades small, adult	Semirigid stylets
Endotracheal tubes, 5.0, 6.0, 7.0, 7.5, 8.0, 8.5 mm	Endotracheal tubes, armored, 7.0, 8.0 mm

Drawer four: LMAs, Combitube

Laryngeal mask airway, no. 3 (small adults)	Intubating laryngeal masks and tubes size 3, 4, 5
Laryngeal mask airway, no. 4 (adults)	Combitube (two)

Drawer five: Retrograde intubation set, transtracheal jet ventilation

Retrograde intubation set	Intravenous angiocatheter 14-gauge
Transtracheal jet ventilation (preassembled)*	Transtracheal catheter, nonkinking

Drawer six: Cricothyrotomy kits

Cricothyrotomy kits (2, preassembled)*	Tracheostomy tubes cuffed, no. 4 Shiley
Commercial percutaneous cricothyrotomy kits	Surgical drapes

Drawer 7: Masks, suction catheters, miscellaneous

Colorimetric end-tidal CO_2 detectors	Endotracheal tube exchangers
Bulb aspiration device (tube detector)	Tracheal suction catheters
Masks	Nasopharyngeal airways, 26, 28, 30, 32, 34 F
Gum elastic bougie	
Wire cutters	Oral airways, 80, 90, 100 mm

*Preparation of a cricothyrotomy kit and a PTTV device is described in Chapter 11.

sive devices from damage and loss. The light source can be attached to the top of the cart without compromising the work surface too much.

ADDITIONAL READING

Caplan RA, Benumof JL, Berry FA, et al. Practice guidelines for the difficult airway: a report by the American Society of Anesthesiologists Task Force on Management of the Difficult Airway. *Anesthesiology* 1993;78:597–602.

The UCSD Department of Anesthesiology has an informative web site which features a "virtual difficult airway cart" at http://www.anesth.ucsd.edu/anesth/Airway/index.html.

MANUFACTURERS LISTING

This is a limited vendor list of manufacturers of emergency airway products. This is by no means complete and does not represent our endorsement of a company or product. Several companies have a web site.

Allegiance Healthcare
V. Meuller division
Surgical instruments
1435 Lake Cook Road
Deerfield, IL 60015
(800) 323-9088; Main: 847-940-5000

Breathing Services, Inc.
931 E. Main Street
POB 817
Ephrata, PA 17522-0817
(717) 733-6579; (800) 732-0028

Ambu, Inc
Intubating heads
611 North Hammonds Ferry Road
Linthicum, MD 21090
(800) 262-8462

Circon ACMI Corp.
Bullard laryngoscope
6500 Hollister Avenue
Santa Barbara, CA 93117
(800) 685-5100; Fax: (805) 968-1265

Anesthesia Associates, Inc.
460 Enterprise Street
San Marcos, CA 92069
(619) 744-6561; Fax: (619) 744-0054

Cook Critical Care
A Division of Cook Incorporated
TTJV catheters, Seldinger cricothyrotomy sets,
   gum elastic bougie, retrograde intubation sets
POB 189
Bloomington, IN 17109
(812) 339-2235; (800) 457-4500
Fax: (800) 554-8335

Armstrong Medical Industries, Inc.
Knightsbridge Parkway
POB 700
Lincolnshire, IL 60069-0700
(800) 323-4220; Fax (847) 913-0138

Heine USA Ltd.
Laryngoscopes
One Washington Street
Unit 555
Dover, NH 03820
(704) 281-8188

Bay Medical, Inc.
13325 US Hwy 19 North
Clearwater, FL 34624
(800) 237-5481; (813) 530-3000
Fax: (813) 531-3991

Instrumentation Industries, Inc.
2990 Industrial Boulevard
Bethel Park, PA 15102-2536
(412) 854-1133; (800) 633-8577
Fax: (412) 854-5668

Kendall Healthcare (Sheridan)
Combitube Airway
(800) 962-9888

Respironics
BL-PAP
(800) 669-9234

Laerdal Medical Corporation
Airway Mgmt Trainers (intubating mannequins)
167 Myers Corners Road
PO Box 1840
Wappingers Falls, NY 12590-8840
(800) 648-1851

Rusch, Inc.
Trachlight lighted stylet
2450 Meadowbrook Parkway
Duluth, GA 30096
(770) 623-0816; (800) 524-7722
Fax: (770) 623-1829

LMA North America
Laryngeal mask airways
9360 Towne Centre Drive
San Diego, CA 92121
(800) 788-7999
Fax: (619) 622-5555

SIMS Portex Inc.
Endotracheal tubes
10 Bowman Drive
POB 0724
Keene, NH 03431
(800) 258-5361

Mercury Medical
TTJV devices, fiberoptic laryngoscope
11300A-49th Street North
Clearwater, FL 34622-4800
(813) 573-0088; (800) 237-6418
Fax: (813) 573-6040

Thompson Dental Company
2422 Devine Street
Columbia, SC 29205
(803) 799-4920; (800) 948-1599
Fax: (803) 771-7351

Nellcor Puritan Bennett, Inc.
Ventilators, BL-PAP, end-tidal CO_2 detectors,
    endotracheal tubes, laryngoscopes, stylets, bags, masks
4280 Hacienda Drive
Pleasanton, CA 94588
(925) 463-4000; (800) 635-5267
Fax: (925) 463-4420

Vital Signs Inc.
20 Campus Road
Totowa, NJ 07512
(800) 932-0760; (973) 790-1330
Fax: (973) 790-3307

Pentax Precision Instrument Corporation
Fiberoptic bronchoscopes
30 Ramland Road
Orangeburg, NY 10962-2699
(914) 365-0700

Xomed
6743 Southpoint Drive, North
Jacksonville, FL 32216-6218
(904) 296-9600; (800) 874-5797
Fax: (904) 281-9735

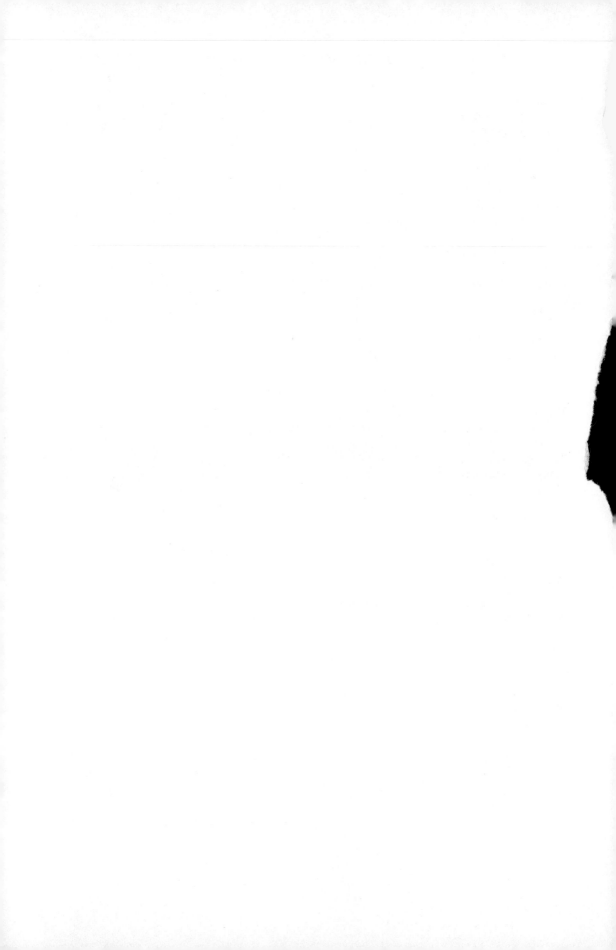

Subject Index

Page number followed by *f* indicates figure, followed by *t* indicates table.

A

Abscess
  peritonsillar, 35
  prevertebral, 35
  retropharyngeal
    in children, 116
Acetylcholinesterase inhibitors
  in competitive nondepolarizing
    NMBA reversal, 126
Acute pulmonary edema,
  175–177
  airway management of,
    175–176
  clinical challenge of, 175
  mechanical ventilation for, 176
  recommended intubation
    sequence for, 176
Adenoids
  in children, 143
Adolescents
  blind NTI in, 110
  Comitube in, 110
  surgical cricothyroidotomy in,
    110–111, 110*f*
Air
  subcutaneous
    during intubation assess-
      ment, 6
Airway
  anatomy of
    in trauma patients, 156
  in children, 57, 143–144, 147*f*,
    148–149
    nasopharyngeal, 148–149
    oral, 148
    oropharyngeal, 56
    shape of, 147*f*
  difficult. *See* Difficult airway
  examination of
    in trauma patients, 154
  failed. *See* Failed airway
  nasopharyngeal, 43, 148–149

  oropharyngeal, 43
  protective reflex of
    evaluation of, 4
  surface anatomy of, 92*f*
Airway intervention
  in children
    timing of, 115–116, 116*t*
Airway maintenance
  failure of
    as intubation indicator, 4
    in prehospital setting, 195
Airway management, 43–57
  intubation in
    anatomy of, 45–46
  laryngoscopy in, 46–56
    nonvisual, 46–51
    paraglossal technique, 46
    tongue control during, 46,
      46*f*
    visual, 49, 54–56
  surgical
    definition of, 89–90
  technique of, 43–45
    BMV evaluation in, 43–44
    head and neck positioning
      in, 43
    jaw position in, 44
    with spontaneous ventilation,
      44–45
    upper airway adjunct
      insertion in, 43
    ventilation assessment in, 45
Airway manager
  role of
    in airway management,
      31–32
Airway obstruction
  and difficult airway prediction,
    33–36
  from foreign bodies, 190–193
Airway protection
  in prehospital setting, 196–197

Airway resistance
  definition of, 211
Albuterol
  for asthma, 164
Algorithms, 16–26
  crash airway. *See* Crash airway
    algorithm
  difficult airway. *See* Difficult
    airway algorithm
  failed airway. *See* Failed airway
    algorithm
  main. *See* Main algorithm
Alpha–adrenergic agents
  for septic shock, 179
Alpha–adrenergic receptor
  blockade, 135
American College of Surgeons'
  Committee on Trauma
  airway management algorithm
    for trauma patients, 16
Amidate, 132. *See also* Etomidate
Aminosteroid compounds, 126
Amyotrophic lateral sclerosis
  and SCh–induced hyper-
    kalemia, 124
Anaphylaxis, 178–179
  airway management of,
    178–179
  clinical challenge of, 178
  mechanical ventilation for, 179
Anatomical landmarks
  in intubation, 45–46
Anectine. *See* Succinylcholine
Anesthesia
  topical
    in difficult airway, 36–37
Anticholinergics
  for COPD, 167–168
Apnea test, 167
Arthritis
  cervical spine, 188
  temporomandibular joint, 188